ORAL PATHOLOGY

ORAL PATHOLOGY

An Introduction to General and Oral Pathology for Hygienists

DONALD A. KERR, B.S., D.D.S., M.S.

Professor of Dentistry; Chairman, Department of Oral Pathology, The University of Michigan School of Dentistry, Ann Arbor, Michigan

MAJOR M. ASH, Jr., B.S., D.D.S., M.S.

Professor of Dentistry; Chairman, Department of Occlusion, The University of Michigan School of Dentistry, Ann Arbor, Michigan

THIRD EDITION

224 Illustrations on 163 Figures

Lea & Febiger • PHILADELPHIA • 1971

First Edition, 1960
Second Edition, 1965
Reprinted December, 1967
Third Edition, 1971

ISBN 0-8121-0339-4

Library of Congress Catalog Card Number 72-135686

Printed in the United States of America

• Preface

As in prior editions this book is intended as an introduction to general and oral pathology for the dental hygienist. The material covered is based on the recognized special needs of the hygienist in relation to her part in total patient care. The title and nature of the contents of the book indicate the significant body of information required for the scope of responsibility enjoyed by the dental hygienist. With the ever-increasing demands for dental care it is obvious that this responsibility is becoming increasingly important and that the science of pathology is becoming one of the most essential prerequisites to clinical practice.

Although the general format of this book remains the same, new and pertinent material has been added to keep abreast of changes in the concepts of disease. In light of an almost explosive increase in knowledge in that part of biology called cell theory, owing to the use of the electron microscope and the work of biochemists, the cellular basis for disease has been expanded. Also, because of recent contributions to genetic theory and disease, a more detailed account of hereditary disease will be found in this edition than in the former editions.

In keeping with the principle that a good illustration can always be improved, many illustrations have been replaced and many new ones added. All references have been reviewed in the light of their contribution to present-day concepts; none have been deleted or added for the sake of having the latest copyright date. Considerable emphasis has been placed on providing at least one or two references in each chapter for the reader who has had little or no training in the basic sciences.

We are greatly indebted to many individuals for assistance in preparation of the third edition. We wish to thank Miss Betty Sundbeck, our secretary, for her assistance; Miss Sally Holden for her suggestions and planning of the revision; Dr. J. Philip Sapp for his suggestions and provision of the ultrastructure photographs; and Mr. Edward Crandell, senior photographer at the School of Dentistry, for preparation of photographs.

DONALD A. KERR
MAJOR M. ASH, JR.

Ann Arbor, Michigan

• Preface to the Second Edition

THE guiding principles for writing the first edition of this book have also served in the preparation of the second edition. These principles include providing an account of the processes of disease, and the essential background for the recognition and prevention of disease within the scope of responsibility and practice of the dental hygienist.

To facilitate the use of this book in the classroom, some revision of the sequence of the material presented has been undertaken. Although the coverage in the first edition proved to be adequate in most respects, it has become apparent that additional topics should be included for those hygienists and students and teachers of dental hygiene who desired more information on specific disease states than was present in the first edition. For these reasons additional chapters on endocrine diseases and blood dyscrasias have been included in the present edition. These chapters have been placed at the end of the text so that they need not be read for a basic concept of disease. This arrangement does not detract from the orderly arrangement of the subject matter since there are references to these chapters in the course of the book and the material may be smoothly incorporated into the basic approach to disease found earlier in the book if desired. The objectives of the second edition have also been emphasized in the additional chapters in that the significance of endocrine and blood diseases has been related to oral disease, especially periodontal disease.

Many areas of the first edition have been revised and expanded to account for recent research and interest. However, the reader and teacher of the first edition will be on familiar ground since the new inclusions have been incorporated largely within the organization of each chapter of the first edition. Because of the importance and emphasis placed on nutrition, the section on malnutrition has been expanded and established as a chapter on Nutritional Disturbances. Although the general manifestations of nutritional deficiencies have been included, the emphasis on oral manifestations has been maintained in light of presently acceptable evidence.

We are greatly indebted to many individuals for assistance in the preparation of the second edition. We wish to thank Miss Betty

Sundbeck, our secretary, for secretarial assistance; Mrs. Ellen Hall, librarian of the School of Dentistry, for library services; and Edward Crandell, senior photographer at the School of Dentistry, for the preparation of the photographs.

DONALD A. KERR

MAJOR M. ASH, JR.

Ann Arbor, Michigan

• Preface to the First Edition

To most hygienists and students and teachers of dental hygiene previously published textbooks of oral and general pathology have represented a formidable coverage of disease unlikely to be encountered as a responsibility of the hygienist in clinical practice. This book has been written especially for the practicing hygienist and the student of dental hygiene to provide a simple and understandable account of the processes of disease and to provide the essential background for the recognition and prevention of diseases within the scope of responsibility and practice of the dental hygienist. An attempt has been made to establish a proper balance between the principles of pathology and the coverage of specific diseases in order to bridge the gap between general pathology and applied oral pathology. Such a balance is possible because the hygienist does not have the responsibility for the diagnosis and treatment of oral disease, and therefore much of the details of diagnosis and treatment of specific diseases found in standard texts of general and oral pathology can be omitted. The omission of such details should not minimize the role of the hygienist in the prevention of disease. The hygienist performs various services in the presence of systemic and oral diseases. These services will be of greater value and more ably carried out if the hygienist understands the principles of pathology. Furthermore the responsibility of the hygienist in the prevention of periodontal disease will be more adequately appreciated, if the hygienist has an understanding of the disease which she is trying to prevent. For example, the hygienist is responsible for the removal of stains, plaque, and calculus from the teeth and as such is as important as any other part of dental practice, since accretions on the teeth are the most important etiologic factors in periodontal disease. In this respect the hygienist is practicing preventive periodontics. Thus a basic understanding of the pathogenesis of accretions is essential for their prevention and removal as well as an understanding of the pathogenesis of periodontal disease.

It is important that the hygienist understand some of the aspects of general pathology; not only as the foundation for its application to the mouth, but as a basis for recognizing those departures of the patient from good health which may have an important bearing on what is done for the patient. For example, scaling procedures may result in a transient bacteremia leading to subacute bacterial endocarditis. An understanding of the relationship between scaling procedures and endocarditis provides the hygienist with an interesting lesson and an enlightened interest in the cause and prevention of disease.

It is hoped that this book will stimulate an interest in pathology and provide an adequate foundation for its appreciation in clinical practice. An appreciation for the processes and prevention of disease by the hygienist is becoming an increasingly important consideration with our rapidly expanding population and failure to keep abreast of the expanding needs of detecting disease. Thus one of the objectives of this book is to provide the foundation for the expanding role of the hygienist in assisting the dentist in the detection and prevention of disease.

We wish to thank those who contributed greatly to the preparation of this text: Mr. Edward Crandell, photographer at the School of Dentistry, for the preparation of the photographs; Miss Rose Grace Faucher, librarian at the School of Dentistry for library services; and Miss Betty Sundbeck, secretary, who contributed many hours of secretarial assistance.

DONALD A. KERR
MAJOR M. ASH, JR.

Ann Arbor, Michigan

• Contents

Chapter 6

Chapter 7

Chapter 8

Chapter 1

INTRODUCTION

DEFINITION OF PATHOLOGY

Pathology is the phase of biology dealing with the causes and mechanisms of disease of all living things. Living things are composed of units called cells that are united in various arrangements to carry out the functions of harmonious and coordinated activity which allow the organism to adapt to its environment and to react to it in a manner suitable for the survival of the species. Cellular activity and reaction to environment are the essence of life. When changes in environment alter the normal response or function of the cells or the organism as a whole the alteration is termed disease. Thus, any change in form or function of the living organism or of its unit parts, so that life exists outside the range of normal, is considered disease. Pathology, then, should be considered the study of life and the attempt to understand life as it exists under abnormal conditions. The aim of pathology is an integrated knowledge of altered form and function. Understanding the interrelationship between altered form and function provides the cornerstone for the study of all the health sciences.

An alteration in form or function of one part of the body may affect the existence of the entire organism or only the part that is altered. This broad scope of pathology requires the investigation and understanding of the interrelationship between the types of alterations in all body areas. On this basis there are many approaches to the study of pathology: it may be *morphologic,* in which alterations in form are emphasized (gross and microscopic pathology); it may be *physiologic,* in which the alterations of function are considered (physiologic pathology); it may be *experimental,* in which attempts are made to investigate the cause of specific alterations, to produce changes previously observed or to find means to prevent or correct tissue alterations (experimental pathology).

Pathology is the study of life outside the range of normal—from death of a few cells to death of the whole body. Disease is always antagonistic to the survival of the organism, and the complete in-

1

ability of the organism to adapt to an unfavorable environment results in its death. A study of pathology is necessary in order to understand the significant alterations in form and function which are considered to be disease and to learn how such alterations may be changed to establish health.

CELLULAR BASIS OF LIFE AND DISEASE

The body is composed of small units called cells. Each cell has a boundary (cell membrane) enclosing a semisolid-like material called the cytoplasm, which contains various organelles, and a more solid body called the nucleus. Although all cells are basically alike, they vary in shape, size, and consistency in various parts of the body, depending on the function they are to perform.

The *cytoplasm* is important in the multiplication of cells, the elimination of waste products, the assimilation and storage of food, and the secretion of enzymes. Within the cytoplasm of most cells is a complicated system of structures called *organelles* (Fig. 1). These internal components of the cell are the plasma membrane, endoplasmic reticulum, ribosomes, mitochondria, Golgi apparatus, lysosomes, centrosome, and centrioles. In addition, inclusions, such as fat, glycogen, proteins, starches, and secretory products, are found in the cytoplasm. The *nucleus* of the cell is concerned primarily with the growth and development of the cell, the metabolic processes inside the cell, the control of reproduction, and the transfer of hereditary

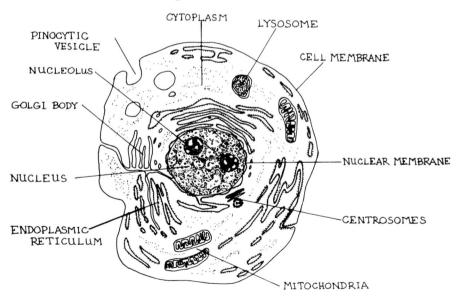

Figure 1. Schematic representation of a cell showing organelles.

characteristics. The *plasma membrane* defines the boundary of the cell and is a dynamic structure of lipoprotein having a highly selective permeability. It is functionally sensitive to the molecular size and biochemical nature of substances as well as to electrical charges. The functional activity of the plasma membrane is important in maintaining the cell as a functional unit and is an essential part of the internal structure of the cell. It is not difficult to appreciate the complexity of the functions of the components of the cell or that disease may be the result of dysfunction of any of the components even at the molecular level. Although Rudolf Virchow, in 1858, changed the concepts of disease by proposing that the cell was not only the unit of life but was also the indivisible unit of disease, it would have been impossible for him to have foreseen the current extension of his concept to cellular subunits.

Of particular interest in periodontal pathology is the nature of the attachment mechanisms among gingival epithelial cells and between the gingival epithelium and the tooth surfaces. Although it is apparent that the attachment apparatus among epithelial cells is in part the desmismose (Fig. 2) and that there is a hemidesmisome-basement lamina complex between the epithelium and the subadjacent connective tissues, the role of the hemidesmisome in the attachment of the gingiva to the tooth is still obscure. The mode of attachment is important in relation to disturbances in the attachment associated with injury to the gingiva (gingivitis) owing to the presence of bacteria, plaque, and calculus on the teeth.

Disturbances in the formation and maintenance of the connective tissue of the periodontal membrane are also of interest in periodontal pathology. The cells that produce the fibers and ground substance of the periodontal membrane are the fibroblasts, which are descended from primitive mesenchymal cells (Fig. 3). The connective tissue, the primary constituent of the periodontal membrane, chiefly is composed of a protein called collagen. The formation of collagen involves the nucleus and ribosomes, which are in contact with and adjacent to the endoplasmic reticulum of the fibroblast. The nucleus initiates the process of collagen formation, but the process is transferred to the ribosomes in the cytoplasm of the cell for continuation. DNA (deoxyribonucleic acid), localized in the nucleus, presides over the synthesis of RNA (ribonucleic acid), which is responsible for the transfer of processing information to the ribosomes. The messenger RNA acts as a template and arranges the proper amino acids into chains, an intermediate process in the formation of collagen. The completion of mature collagen and its formation into functional fibers in the periodontal membrane are completed outside of the cell. A disturbance in the process can result in disease; for example,

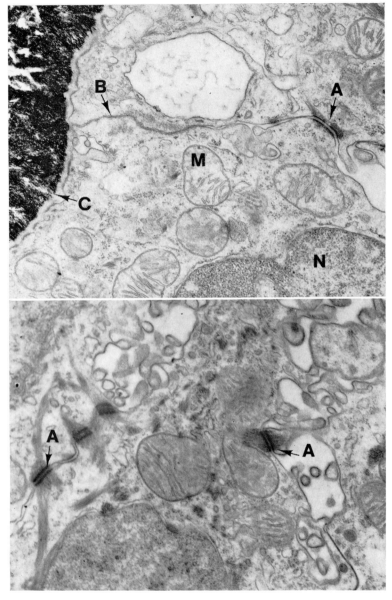

Figure 2. *Upper, Ultrastructure of an odontogenic cell.* Desmisome (A), cell
membranes of adjacent cells (B), outer surface of tooth (C), mitochondria (M), nucleus of cell (N). *Lower,* There are four desmisomes (A) present in the part of the cell represented. Two of the
four desmisomes are indicated.

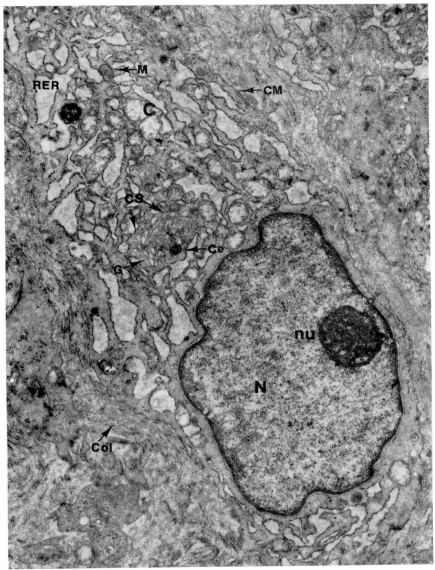

Figure 3. *Ultrastructure of a differentiating cell.* The nucleus (N) contains a prominent eccentrically placed nucleolus (nu). The cytoplasm (C) contains dilated, rough endoplasmic reticulum (RER) and mitochondria (M). Since the section is through the center of the cell, the centrosphere area (CS) is present and demonstrates the Golgi apparatus (G) and a cross section through one of the centrioles (Ce). The cell is contained by the cytoplasmic membrane (CM). Strands and bundles of collagen fibers (Col) are found adjacent to the cytoplasmic membrane. Magnification approximately × 12,240.

a deficiency of vitamin C interferes with the intermediate process of collagen formation and results in scurvy. Of particular importance in the study of the initiation and progress of periodontal disease is the production of hyaluronidase by bacteria in dental plaque on teeth. Proteolytic enzymes are capable of breaking down the collagen fibers in the periodontal membrane resulting in a loss of the supporting structures of the teeth. Disturbances in the formation and maintenance of the connective tissues are important in many diseases including inherited disorders and disturbances of the joints, such as rheumatoid arthritis.

Lysosomes, which are confined in vacuoles in cells, contain enzymes capable of the "digestion" of bacteria and other particulate matter engulfed by the cells. These enzymes are also involved in the breakdown of dead cells. Lysosomes are most prominent in cells capable of ingestion of bacteria and other particles (phagocytosis), but may be found in additional cells as well. Cells capable of phagocytosis include certain white blood cells (polymorphonuclear leukocytes), which are important in the defense of the body against infection (see Fig. 46).

The process of cell division (mitosis), whereby growth and reproduction are made possible, is a function of the nucleus. Previous to cell division, the nucleus contains a granular material called chromatin, which becomes incorporated into small strands called chromosomes as cell division begins. Chromosomes contain the elements that dictate the character of the cells. In the sex cells the chromosomes are the structures which transmit genetic factors from the parent to his offspring, and thus are responsible for the transmission of certain features from the parent to his offspring. These transmitted features are called hereditary features. In the process of cell division the chromatin is incorporated into and replaced by chromosomes, which divide longitudinally into a set number of rod-like chromosomes. One-half of the chromosomes moves to one side of the cell and one-half moves to the opposite side; then a constriction through the middle divides the cell into two identical cells. It is by this process of cell multiplication that organs increase in size and the body grows. After a part of the body or tissue reaches maturity, the rate of cell division decreases and the part ceases to grow. However, the ability of the cell to divide is retained and can be stimulated to take place when the need arises for new cells to replace areas of injured tissue.

Irritability is the feature of the cell enabling it to respond to various stimuli. Because of the basic property of irritability, proper stimuli may cause a muscle cell to contract, a salivary gland cell to secrete saliva, or a nerve cell to conduct nervous impulses. Nervous tissue has the most advanced development of the property of irritability.

Reactivity, or specificity, is the property of a cell to respond specifically to a stimulus. It is the ability of a cell to carry out a specific function as determined by the structure of the cell. Such cells have no capacity to alter their specific functions and can only reproduce the same type of specialized cell. The cytoplasm of the cell is chiefly responsible for this functional activity. *Absorption* is the process of taking dissolved substance into the cell. This physiologic property of the protoplasm of a cell enables it to obtain the necessary materials for its function. *Excretion* is the ability of a cell or group of cells to eliminate waste products from within the cell or body. *Secretion* refers to the ability of a cell or group of cells to elaborate a specific product for use locally or for the whole organism: for example, the parotid glands are groups of cells elaborating saliva; the thyroid gland produces hormones for the whole organism.

Cells are formed into groups or systems having a particular architectural characteristic for each organ or tissue. Thus one or more aggregates of cells, all having the same function and morphologic characteristics, form the liver, another group muscles, another bone, and another nerve tissue. The grouping of specialized cells for the purpose of special functions represents a high degree of development of the physiologic properties of individual cells, i.e., absorption by intestines, excretion by kidneys, secretion by adrenal glands, assimilation by liver, and conduction by nerves. This state of development and specialization of cells makes all cells and aggregrates of cells dependent upon each other to a certain degree. Such dependence is of some disadvantage to the organism, since an alteration of function in one area may upset the function of cells in another area. Thus, all cells function as individual units and as groups for the advantage of the whole body. Any alteration of one or more of the aggregates of cells may jeopardize the efforts of a whole community of cells or of the whole organism itself. For example, the injury and destruction of only a certain area of muscle cells of the heart may cause the heart to stop functioning and cause the death of the organism. The regulation and integration of cells functioning for the welfare of the whole organism are based on activities of the blood-vascular system, the nervous system, and the endocrine glands.

One additional fact should be considered in visualizing the alteration of cellular life as the basis of disease *(cellular pathology)*: intercellular substances, which are formed by the cells, are responsible for the continuity that exists among cells and give the cells and organism support. Thus, intercellular substances are intimately related to the health of the cells and the organism.

All cells are interrelated with other cells of the body because of the media in which they exist. Each individual cell is composed largely of fluid and is bathed in fluid. The wall of the cell is permeable so fluid elements may pass from the cell into the surrounding media and so fluids from the environment of the cell can pass into the cell (Fig. 4). In this manner cells obtain the metabolic materials they need to remain alive and to function, and pass the waste products of cell metabolism into the environmental fluid. In order that food materials may be brought to the environment of the cells and that waste products may be carried away, another fluid system exists—the blood-vascular system. The blood-vascular system is a closed tubular system for the circulation of fluid to cells throughout the body. The walls of this tubular system, like the cell membrane, are permeable; fluids pass through them into the spaces between the cells, and fluid from the intercellular spaces pass into blood and lymph vessels. The interchange between tissue fluid and blood permits transportation of materials from one area of the body to another and permits the products of a cell to be transported to another part of the body for utilization by other cells. Thus, it is through this fluid medium and its circulation that a single organ influences all the cells of the body (Fig. 5). When this interchange functions properly, it is for the good of the entire community of cells and results in health; when the function is abnormal, the substances formed may adversely affect certain other cells in the community

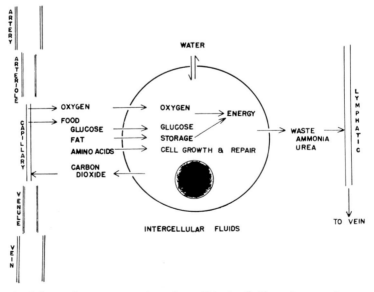

Figure 4. Schematic representation of a cell in its fluid environment.

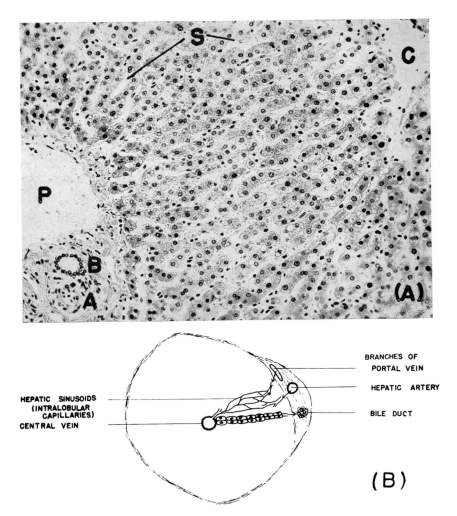

Figure 5. (A), *Liver lobule*. P, B, and A make up the portal canal. Branch of portal vein, P; bile duct, B; hepatic arteriole, A; central vein C; sinusoids, S. (B), Diagram of entire liver lobule.

and disease results, or when severe enough, they cause the death of the entire body.

As the cells function in their fluid environment, substances may be carried to the cells that are toxic and cause the death of a few cells. Dead cells are replaced by new ones produced by division of the remaining cells. Thus tissues are made up of cells of varying ages. As the organism ages, the process of maintaining suitable living conditions within the fluid environment becomes increasingly diffi-cult for the following reasons: the intercellular substance seems to deteriorate with age and is not efficiently or effectively replaced; the cells react to stimuli more slowly and less effectively; and the body and all its parts undergo degenerative changes. These changes are called aging, a retrogressive process starting at birth and contin-uing until cell life cannot be maintained and death results. Between these two extremes there may be numerous alterations in one or more parts of the body that are not directed toward maintaining the general welfare of the entire body. The alteration of cells in-volved in the maintenance of a part of the organism represents dis-ease of that part. It is the alterations in structure and function of cellular units that constitute disease—the subject that pathology treats.

SUMMARY

The cells of a complex organism, such as the human body, have the ability to react individually or as an aggregate to environmental changes that affect the whole organism. These reactions, "cellular altruism," help the individual to survive in his environment.

Because of the intimate relationship of cells existing in a common fluid media, environmental changes affecting one cell will affect many cells in the same area. Thus, the way in which a cell responds to changes in environment is determined in part by the type of alteration which occurs in the fluid environment. In addition, the continuity of cellular environment provided by the fluid media and blood-vascular system permits changes in one area to influence changes in another area of the body. This feature of cellular inte-gration may be desirable or undesirable as far as the entire organism is concerned. It is desirable as far as integration of nutrition, func-tion, and communication are concerned, but undesirable if the natural barriers to the spread of injurious agents are not operating effectively.

The foregoing discussion has provided the reader with the follow-ing concepts: (1) life and disease are inseparable because disease merely represents life outside of the range of normal; (2) the cellu-lar basis of life is also the basis of cellular reactions to disease or injury; (3) disease represents a state of life disadvantageous to the whole organism; and (4) health is life within the range of normal and advantageous to the continuation of the human species. Finally, the study and understanding of pathology are necessary prerequi-sites for individuals who wish to restore tissue to a healthy state and to prevent disease.

BIBLIOGRAPHY

Anderson, W. A. D.: *Pathology*. St. Louis, The C. V. Mosby Company, 1966, Chapter One.

Bender, G. A.: Virchow and cellular pathology. Therap. Notes, 68:149, 1961.

Kennedy, D.: *The Living Cell*. Scientific American Ed. San Francisco and London, W. H. Freeman and Co., 1965.

Listgarten, M. A.: The ultrastructure of human gingival epithelium. Amer. J. Anat., 114:49, 1964.

Schroeder, H. E.: Ultrastructure of the junctional epithelium of the human gingiva. Helv. Odont. Acta, 13:65, 1969.

Thilander, H., and Bloom, G. D.: Cell contacts in oral epithelium. J. Periodont. Res., 3:96, 1968.

Chapter 2

CAUSES AND MECHANISMS OF DISEASE

Disease is produced by a wide variety of etiologic factors which can be divided into three groups: (1) intrinsic factors, (2) extrinsic factors, and (3) developmental factors. Although each of these causative factors is responsible respectively for intrinsic disease, extrinsic disease, and developmental disease, each factor acts in a different manner and at a different time to produce disease. The causes of disease enumerated above will be enlarged upon to demonstrate the part each plays in the production of disease.

INTRINSIC FACTORS

Diseases that involve changes in the germ plasm are called intrinsic diseases, and the etiologic factors responsible for the production of these diseases are intrinsic factors. The intrinsic factors for the transmission of disease are contained within the chromosomes of the sex cells and are called genes. When a gene for a specific alteration in the form or function of a part is transmitted from one individual to his offspring, the disease is said to be hereditary and the cause intrinsic. Thus intrinsic causative factors are in the cells of the organism and are transmitted by its chromosomes to succeeding generations.

The size, stature, complexion, and function of various parts of an organism are determined by factors transmitted in the germ plasm. They are the normal characteristics of the species and are responsible for the individuality of the organism. However, certain defects may be transmitted in the same manner, and the offspring will exhibit the same defect as his parent. This is inherited disease, and the factor responsible for its development is an intrinsic factor. Hereditary diseases are transmitted through the germ plasm by factors contained in the chromosomes.

There are many factors for disease which are transmitted by the germ plasm. Examples of inheritable diseases are color blindness, hemophilia, albinism, absence of parts (failure of teeth, toes, or fingers to develop), and the tendency to develop neoplasia, diabetes, and certain types of insanity. Color blindness is a hereditary disease said to be sex linked because the genes responsible for transmitting color blindness are in the chromosome that determines sex. The factor for color blindness is in the chromosomes dictating that the individual is to be a male; therefore color blindness is present in men. The disease is transmitted from the affected grandfather through the unaffected daughter to the grandson. Several disease processes demonstrate this pattern of sex-linked inheritance; one of a very severe nature is hemophilia. The hemophilic individual lacks the mechanism for controlling hemorrhage so with minor injuries resulting in bleeding, the uncontrolled hemorrhage may cause death.

Disturbances in the formation of enamel (amelogenesis imperfecta) and disturbances in the formation of dentin (dentinogenesis imperfecta) are dominant hereditary conditions. Dominance means that the trait will appear in several members of every generation. These diseases are discussed under disturbances in the development of teeth on pages 57, 62.

Congenital absence of teeth is intrinsic in character, either as an individual trait or as part of a syndrome, such as anhidrotic ectodermal dysplasia in which the individual fails to develop hair, sweat glands, and sebaceous glands. Sometimes there is failure to develop nails, and many of the individuals affected have very few or no teeth.

There are many syndromes in which oral alterations are a part of the picture of inherited diseases. They may involve too few or too many teeth, alteration in palatal and mandibular forms, and changes in the oral mucosa. Some inheritable disturbances are enamel hypoplasia, dentin dysplasia, hare lip, cleft palate, and hereditary gingival fibromatosis. These conditions are discussed under developmental disturbances in Chapter Three.

Lack or abnormal development of fingers and toes is an inheritable abnormality. Extra fingers and toes (polydactyl) and webbed fingers and toes (syndactyl) are family traits. Hair and eye colors are determined by hereditary factors, brown eyes being dominant over blue.

Individuals also inherit certain patterns of endocrine gland activity and metabolism. Deficiencies in these patterns of gland function and metabolism, which the individual inherits, predispose him to the development of specific diseases. The individual may inherit the tendency for the development of diabetes, gout, or tuberculosis; the disease is not inherited, but the constitution that makes the individual prone to develop the disease is inherited. Other diseases of intrinsic character are discussed in appropriate locations throughout the text.

Genetic Principles

Until recently most of the concepts of genetics were based on observations of the effect of selective breeding and on chromosome mechanics during cell division. The transmission of genes from one generation to another was considered to be the result of certain characteristics in the sperm and egg. Such characteristics are contained within the chromosomes derived from each parent. If the genes at a given point on each of the paired chromosomes are identical, the person is said to be *homozygous* for the trait provided by the genes. If the genes are unlike in their responsibility for a particular trait, the individual is said to be *heterozygous* for the specified trait. If one of the two determinants of a trait is expressed in the characteristics of the offspring and the other is not, the expressed determinant is *dominant* and the nonexpressed determinant *recessive*. Two other terms in general use in genetics are *genotype,* meaning genetic constitution, and *phenotype,* meaning the appearance of an individual (more specifically that appearance resulting from the interaction of environment on the genotype). At this point it is obvious that most of the genetic concepts expressed provide for the recognition of hereditary disease and, to some extent, to relate the disease to specific chromosomes. However, with the extensive growth of knowledge about the biochemical processes involved in cellular and genetic functions, it is now possible to obtain a better understanding of the way a gene determines a particular characteristic. With the union of the classical concepts of genetics and the chemical basis for inheritance, the pathology of inherited diseases has been greatly expanded.

A key to the control of genetic processes is the biochemical structure of the chromosomes. The chromosome consists of numerous strands of DNA (deoxyribonucleic acid), a giant molecule. Genetic information is stored in the DNA molecule in the form of a code. The information stored in the code is transmitted from the DNA of the gene to a particular type of RNA (ribonucleic acid) or messenger RNA. The messenger RNA transfers the genetic information from the nucleus to the ribosomes in the cytoplasm. The ribosomes are active in protein synthesis and the messenger RNA acts as a template for the correct assembling of amino acids in sequence. While an oversimplification of the process has been stated, the DNA molecule can reproduce itself into two exact copies and pass the genetic code from one generation to another. The genetic code essentially consists of code letters in the DNA molecule made up of four bases or subunits, adenine, guanine, cytosine, and thymine. Various combinations of these code letters, or nucleotide bases, provide the biochemical information used by the cell for the construction of proteins. Proteins are large molecules constructed from 20 amino acids. The giant molecules, consisting of chains of various amino acids, are formed according to the sequence of the letters in the inherited DNA molecule(s). Thus the code specifies the proper amino acid and its location in the chain of amino acids making up the protein.

At first the problem of a genetic code centered around the question of how a four-letter alphabet (the bases or subunits) could specify a 20-word dictionary corresponding to 20 amino acids. It is generally held at the present time that the genetic information stored in the DNA molecule is in the form of a triplet code, i.e., a sequence of three bases determine the structure of one amino acid. Thus, if three bases specify one amino acid, the possible combinations of four bases taken three at a time would be 64. This number is more than enough to account for the 20 amino acids.

Inborn Errors of Metabolism

The relationship between genes and protein synthesis is apparent when a cellular defect alters the control of a biologic process. Since a metabolic process proceeds by steps and each step is controlled by a specific enzyme, an interference with one of the steps may result from the failure of a gene to produce the enzyme properly. Examples of this problem include phenylketonuria, albinism, and alkaptonuria. In individuals with phenylketonuria the enzyme necessary for the conversion of phenylalanine to tyrosine is deficient. With the accumulation of phenylalanine there is damage to the central nervous system resulting in severe mental retardation.

If the enzyme defect results in a deficiency of products normally formed as a result of the enzyme, a disease such as hypophosphatasia may occur. In hypophosphatasic patients, rachitic-like bone lesions occur and often teeth are lost from severe periodontal disease.

Certain inborn errors of metabolism are due to an accumulation of metabolic products not acted upon by a deficient enzyme. If the products are of large molecular size a storage disease may occur, such as gargoylism, congenital porphyria, or Gaucher's disease. There are structural oral defects in gargoylism, and intrinsic staining of the teeth in congenital porphyria.

Chromosomes and Abnormalities

Genetic abnormalities may be the result of failure in chromosome mechanics at some point, viz., reduction in the number of chromosomes from the diploid to the haploid number (meiosis). In man there are a total of 46 chromosomes in the normal somatic cell, but in meiosis there is a reduction from the haploid number of 46 to the diploid number of 23. Alterations in the number and/or structure of either the sex or autosomal chromosomes can result in clinically recognizable disease.

A well-known disorder involving an extra autosomal chromosome is mongolism. Patients with the disease usually have 47 chromosomes. Mongoloid children often are mentally retarded, develop characteristic facial and head appearance, die young, and have an increased susceptibility to infection, including a form of ulcerative necrotizing gingivitis. Some forms of mongolism do not involve an extra chromosome but rather are due to a structural defect (translocation) in chromosomes.

There are one-half as many chromosomes in the nuclei of sex cells (gametes) as there are in nuclei of body (somatic) cells. In man the 22 pairs of chromosomes in the somatic cells are autosomes or autosomal chromosomes. The remaining two pair are sex chromosomes and are termed X and Y chromosomes. In men one X chromosome and one Y chromosome are present so that males are said to have XY sex chromosome constitutions. In women the sex chromosomes are the same; therefore females have XX sex chromosome constitutions. Each ovum carries one of the X chromosomes, but the sperm may carry either an X or a Y chromosome.

Abnormalities in sex chromosomes are usually related to characteristics which make up the gender of an individual. An individual with an XXY sex chromosome constitution is sterile and often mentally retarded. Apparently there is a relationship between an increased number of X chromosomes and mental retardation. When only one sex chromosome is present in a female (XO sex chromosome constitution) she is sterile and often has congenital abnormalities. Another abnormality is true hermaphroditism in which there is some ambiguity regarding the sexual status of the affected individual.

Inheritance of Traits

Certain diseases appear to affect the members of a family through many generations. Since most diseases do not follow a simple pattern of inheritance, and environmental factors play a significant role in congenital anomalies, it is not always possible to determine whether a certain defect is an inherited trait or not. Observation of the trait in several families over two or three generations may provide sufficient information to determine how the trait is inherited. Several mechanisms for the transmission of traits are possible.

An inherited trait determined by a sex chromosome is considered to be sex linked. A trait determined by a gene on an autosome is

3

inherited as an autosomal trait. Autosomal and sex-linked traits may be dominant or recessive.

In autosomal dominant inheritance one of the parents of the affected individual also has the trait and the abnormal gene which causes the disorder. This is true except in those cases where the parent was affected very mildly and the trait was not apparent, or the trait arose because of a new gene mutation. If an affected individual marries a normal individual, one-half of their children will be affected (assuming sufficient births occur so that an average of one-half is possible). By chance, an affected individual may have all normal or all affected children. Furthermore, the degree of expression of the autosomal dominant trait is quite variable, and in some instances may not be manifest at all in one generation. For example, skeletal and dental defects may be expressed so mildly in osteogenesis imperfecta that their presence may virtually go undetected.

Autosomal recessive traits are only manifested when two genes for the trait or defect are present. Since this possibility is not great most recessive traits are uncommon. The most common recessive defect in man is fibrocystic disease of the pancreas. It occurs once in about 2,000 births. The most uncommon recessive defects are seen most often when there is increased consanguinity among the parents of the affected persons, viz., frequent marriages between first cousins. Of interest in periodontal pathology is the severe precocious periodontitis in palmoplantar hyperkeratosis.

Sex-linked inheritance indicates that the abnormal gene for a defect is carried on the sex chromosome. The defect is manifested in the female only when both genes from the parent are mutant genes for the defect. In the male the defect is almost always manifested, since the mutant gene is carried on a single X chromosome. Diseases of this type are transmitted by normal female carriers and by affected males. An example of a sex-linked recessive trait is hemophilia in which a deficiency of factor VIII (p. 292) causes a defect in blood clotting.

Most of what has been related to inheritance in the foregoing discussion does not take into consideration genetic traits based on multiple alleles (allele refers to alternate forms of a gene occurring at the same point or locus on homologous chromosomes). For example in blood types there are four alleles in the ABO classification, and a person may have any two of the four alleles, viz., AB, OO, and so on. It is apparent that an inherited trait may be the result of a single gene or the modification of a gene by other genes (multifactorial inheritance). Such characteristics as height, weight, skin color, and intelligence are the result of multifactorial inheritance.

Inherited diseases may be due to dominant or recessive genes; however environmental factors, or nonmendelian genetic implications, must also be considered. Genetically determined defects without demonstrable chromosome aberrations include such diseases as osteogenesis imperfecta, multiple polyposis of colon, and multiple exostoses, all of which may have oral manifestations and are examples of autosomal dominant inheritance. In contrast are diseases such as cleft palate, cleft lip, congenital heart disease, diabetes mellitus, peptic ulcer, and tuberculosis which involve not only genetic factors but also, to varying degrees, nonmendelian or environmental influences. In tuberculosis the susceptibility for the disease is inherited, but genetically predisposed individuals in general do not develop the disease unless unfavorable environmental conditions are also present. Similarly, peptic ulcer is more common in children of parents with the disturbance than in children of normal parents, but it does not occur to the same extent without the presence of environmental stress.

Radiation and Heredity

Ionizing radiations that cause damage to the germ plasm include X rays, gamma rays, and high-energy particles such as alpha and beta particles. The amount of radiation absorbed by the tissues is measured in *rads*. If the whole human body is irradiated with a dose of 300 to 500 rads, the dose is usually fatal. Much larger doses are used in the treatment of certain types of tumors, but the dosage involves only a small volume of tissue. The term *rem* is used to indicate the equivalent biologic effect that results from irradiation other than X rays. Thus 1 rem produces the same biologic effect as 1 rad. Since man is exposed to a mixture of radiations, the term rem may be used to compare the amounts of different types of radiation.

The sources of radiation may be natural (cosmic rays and gamma radiation) or artificial (medical and dental radiology, radioactive fallout). It has been calculated that the average gonadal dose from all sources of radiation in 30 years is about 4 rems. The maximum permissible dose of radiation, in addition to natural background radiation (about 3 rems for 30 years), is 5 rems over a period of 30 years.

It has been shown experimentally in plants and animals that mutations are produced in proportion to the dosage of radiation. In addition, the genetic effects of radiation are cumulative. Thus each new dose must be added to previous doses of radiation, the total number of mutations being directly proportional to the total gonadal dosage. Since man receives only about 3 rems of radiation from natural sources over a 30-year period, it appears that the majority (97 percent) of spontaneous mutations must be due to causes other than those from natural sources of radiation.

Of particular interest in assessing the genetic effects of radiation in man is the analysis of births related to parents exposed to atomic radiation at the time of the Nagasaki and Hiroshima bombings. An analysis of several thousands of births showed no significant increase in the incidence of birth defects or stillbirths. Although the vast majority of mutations are harmful and have been shown to occur in plants and animals exposed to radiation, there is no convincing evidence that radiation causes genetic damage in man, at least to immediately involved generations. However, there could well be a hazard to future generations, but more information is necessary before the exact genetic effects of radiation in man can be determined.

EXTRINSIC FACTORS

Extrinsic diseases are produced by etiologic factors brought to the cell from its environment rather than by transmission through chromosomes. Extrinsic factors may be considered as environmental factors if we think of environment in its broad sense—the environment of the individual cell as well as the environment of the organism as a whole. The extrinsic factors producing disease are more numerous than intrinsic factors and therefore are demonstrated more often in relation to disease.

Since oxygen, heat, water, and food are fundamental needs of the body, it is appropriate to consider any alteration of the optimal quantities of these body requirements as extrinsic etiologic factors in causing disease. Physical, chemical, thermal irradiation, microorganisms, and psychologic alterations are also extrinsic factors in the causation of disease.

Oxygen

If the atmosphere is replaced by some other material such as earth or water, the individual is prevented from obtaining oxygen and death results. When an individual is submerged in water, death is due to drowning, but if submerged in sand, death is due to suffocation. The individual may be deprived of oxygen if the air is replaced by another gas as sometimes occurs in deep wells or mines. If the air contains a high concentration of gas for which the hemoglobin has a marked affinity, it replaces the oxygen in the blood stream. An excellent example is carbon monoxide. Hemoglobin has several times the affinity for carbon monoxide than it has for oxygen, so when small quantities are present in the atmosphere, it is absorbed by the hemoglobin and prevents oxygen from being absorbed. The individual cells are thus deprived of oxygen and death is attributed to carbon monoxide poisoning (asphyxiation). Death by asphyxiation occurs when individuals are trapped in smoke-filled rooms during a fire or stay in a closed garage while the car motor is running. Other substances for which hemoglobin demonstrates an affinity may combine with hemoglobin to form a stable chemical compound such as methemoglobin. Methemoglobin, produced in analine poisoning and many other chemical intoxications, does not have an affinity for oxygen and is incapable of transporting oxygen to and from the cells. Although the mechanism of oxygen deficiency associated with methemoglobin is different from low-oxygen tension in the atmosphere or carbon monoxide poisoning, the effect on the cell is the same. Some toxic agents damage and destroy the red blood cells which results in oxygen deficiency and death of the cells.

Cells of a limited area may die because of being deprived of oxygen and nutrients when the blood vessels to the area are obstructed. The local death of cells in a limited area of the body is designated *necrosis,* while the loss of the blood supply to the area leading to the

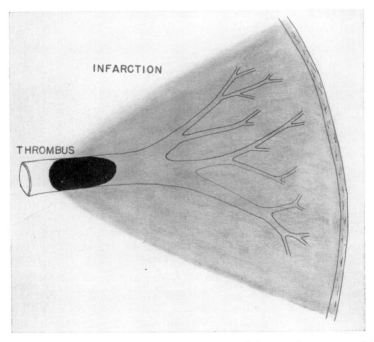

Figure 6. Diagram demonstrating a thrombus and the resultant zone of infarction that might be produced by obstruction of a renal vessel.

death of the cells is called *ischemia*. The process of obstruction of an end-artery or the sole vein of an area and the resulting ischemic necrosis of the area is called *infarction*. The area of tissue that undergoes necrosis is called an infarct (Fig. 6). Obstruction of a vessel may occur as a result of thrombosis or embolism. *Thrombosis* is the intravascular clotting of blood. Most frequently it refers to the formation of a clot within a vessel owing to injury of the endothelial lining; such a clot is referred to as a thrombus. *Embolism* is the transportation of a substance or mass through vessels from one location to a second where it lodges. The mass is referred to as an *embolus*. The most common source of emboli are thrombi which become detached. Thrombosis is significant because of the possibility of occluding the vessels of vital tissues and organs of the body such as the heart. An individual is said to die of a "heart attack" or "coronary" if the coronary vessels of the heart are obstructed or occluded, and the heart muscle dies because of a lack of oxygen and other blood nutrients.

Clinical manifestations of a lack of oxygen (anoxia) are shortness of breath (dyspnea), difficulty in breathing, and deep and rapid breathing. Cyanosis may also be present and is due to an absolute increase in the amount of reduced hemoglobin in the blood. Cyanosis causes the skin and mucous membranes to be dusky blue color. The most common cause of generalized cyanosis is heart disease. Localized cyanosis, which is seen in gingivitis, is primarily due to local changes in circulation (venous congestion or passive hyperemia). *Passive hyperemia* refers to a decreased outflow or a stagnation of blood on the venous side of the circulation. An area so involved is not able to obtain its optimal requirements of oxygen and food. Venous congestion is a common feature of gingivitis. *Active hyperemia* refers to an increased flow of blood to the tissues and in part is responsible for increased heat and redness in inflammation.

Heat

Extremes of temperature, both heat and lack of heat (cold), produce tissue injury. The local application of rather mild heat to the skin causes a moderate increase in temperature resulting in redness and tenderness of the area to which the heat is applied. More intense heat results in the local accumulation of fluid within the tissues beneath the skin. The fluid causes a separation of the tissues and a thinning of the epithelium which results in a blister. If the heat is intense enough, it produces destruction of cells by coagulation of the cytoplasm or by actually burning and charring the tissues. An increase in the environmental temperature for long periods produces heat exhaustion because of the loss of chlorides through excessive perspiration. If the environmental temperature is high and water is unavailable, death from dehydration occurs in a short time.

The effects of cold are similar to those of heat. A mild reduction of temperature results in redness and swelling of the part (frostbite). Further reduction of temperature produces ice crystals which, on thawing, cause blisters in the tissues. If the temperature of a part of the body is reduced to a point where the blood vessels are injured so that the flow of blood into the part ceases, a clot forms within the blood vessels. The blood flow will not return to the part when the temperature returns to normal and the part dies (gangrene). General reduction of body temperature for prolonged periods results in gradual reduction of cell metabolism and death.

Water

Water, as an extrinsic cause of disease, is related to either too much or too little for the requirements of the body. Injury from too much water occurs only rarely, and then it is probably accidental in relation to intravenous or subcutaneous therapy. Insufficient water or excessive loss of water leads to dehydration. An individual may be dehydrated from excessive loss of water, from diarrhea, or from deprivation of water owing to insufficient intake. Infants or children who are sick may reject water or fluids and dehydration occurs. If dehydration progresses, death ensues.

Food

Nutrition is the summation of the dietary intake of food and its absorption, storage, and utilization by the tissues. Disturbances in nutrition result in a variety of disease processes, each having characteristic features and significance. Starvation results when the dietary intake does not meet the nutritional requirements of the individual. A deficient intake of food is compensated by utilization of the fat stored in the fat deposits of the body. After the fat is completely depleted, other tissues are utilized. The loss of fat and other materials causes a reduction in the weight and size of the individual. When the process is severe and all reserves are depleted, death results from starvation. An excess of food causes obesity.

There may be a deficiency in specific food fractions, such as proteins, carbohydrates, and fats. Each type of deficiency produces a specific type of tissue response. An individual who is deficient in protein has poor healing power, because protein is necessary to build new tissue. In addition to the essential food factors, the individual may be deficient in accessory food factors, the most important of which are vitamins. Vitamins are a complex group of substances in food which are necessary for proper cell function. The most important vitamins are A, B, C, and D. (See Nutritional Diseases, Chapter 7, p. 156.)

Mechanical Injury

Mechanical force is a very common cause of tissue injury. Its effects depend upon the site, intensity, and method of application. Tissue or parts may be crushed, torn, and/or abraded; bones may be fractured by mechanical or physical force. Injury produced by physical force is called *trauma*.

The injury produced by mechanical force depends on the area of the body to which the force is applied, the degree of the force, the method of application, and the duration of application. When a force is slight and tangentially applied, it may cause a shallow loss of skin or mucous membrane resulting in a wound called an *abrasion*. *Lacerations* are wounds with jagged margins produced by an irregularly shaped, hard object or by tearing of the tissues. When the physical trauma is produced by a sharp instrument, and the resulting wound has a smooth border, it is called an incisional wound or *incision*. Thin, sharp objects forced into the tissues produce *penetrating* wounds. A bullet may make a penetrating wound, or a perforating wound if it comes out the other side of the body forming two openings. *Contusions* or *bruises* are the result of forces applied by blunt objects which usually do not break the surface of the body but disrupt underlying tissues, viscera, or organs. A bruise is produced when soft tissue is impinged between two hard objects so that the blood vessels are injured and blood escapes into the tissues. This type of physical trauma results in a rather characteristic discoloration of the tissues, "black-and-blue" mark or "black eye." Similarly, a blow to the trunk of the body may rupture and bruise solid viscera like liver or spleen, or hollow viscera like the bladder or gut. Compressive forces produce the same results. Fractures of bones are produced by the sudden application of moderate or severe forces. Fractures vary in pattern, depending upon the area involved and the degree of force. When there is much displacement of the bone fragments and loss of continuity of soft tissue with exposure of bone, the injury is called a *compound fracture*. Microorganisms are frequently introduced into the tissue during mechanical injury producing infection which complicates the process of repair. (See Mechanical Injury, Chapter 12, p. 245.)

Chemical Injury

Injury by chemical substance may occur at the point of application (chemical burns) or the chemical may be carried to all parts of the body and produce injury (poisoning) of a part or all of the body cells. Chemical burns are produced on skin and mucous membrane by the application of toxic materials such as phenol, silver nitrate, acids, strong bases (lye), and many other substances. The lesions produced may be areas of redness, blisters, or ulcers, depending upon the concentration of the chemical, its toxicity, and the length of time it was applied. Toxic substances enter the body by ingestion, injection, absorption, or inhalation and are transported to the cells by the blood. In this way many substances affect selected cells, organs, or the entire body and the effects are designated poisoning.

Toxic substances ingested or injected into the body produce effects locally or systemically as the result of their transportation by the blood to the cells. The most commonly injected poisons are from insect bites. The toxic material entering the tissue in the area of an insect bite is small in quantity but high in toxicity. The toxin from the insect produces a local reaction manifested as redness, swelling, and itching or pain. If larger quantities are introduced into the tissue, as in reptile bites, or if the toxin is potent, as in bites from black widow spiders, the effects are more widespread and death may result.

Toxic substances may be ingested and produce effects in the stomach resulting in nausea and vomiting, which eliminates the poison from the body. If the chemical substance does not produce vomiting, it may be absorbed into the blood and transported to cells. Some substances have a greater affinity for one tissue than for another and the effect produced is dependent upon the tissue affected, viz., some toxins are neurotoxins (coral snake venom and botulinal toxins), others are hemotoxins (rattlesnake venom). Poisons may be produced by microorganisms and have effects comparable to those produced by other chemicals. The bacterial toxins may produce gastric effects as in food poisoning (botulism) or the effects may be general as in diphtheria, tetanus, and other infections. The general effects of poisons are due to changes in the blood cells, the central nervous system, or vital organs.

Chemical substances injurious to the cells may be produced within the body or may enter from the outside. Many of the chemical substances produced by the body are toxic when present in too high a concentration or when in an area where they are not normally present. For example, if the fluid elaborated by the stomach escapes into the abdominal cavity, digestion of tissue occurs although no such effect to the lining of the stomach occurs. (See Chemical Injury, Chapter 12, p. 249.)

Irradiation

Irradiation by radiant energy may occur in several ways, the most common method is exposure to the rays of ultraviolet light or sunlight. These rays penetrate the skin, and when the exposure is intense and of sufficient duration tissue injury results. The initial changes are redness and slight swelling of the area, followed by blister formation if the exposure is intense and prolonged. The pigment of the skin provides some protection against irradiation by sunlight when exposure is not sufficient to produce injury. By repeated minimal exposure, the skin pigment is increased (tanning) providing protection so that greater exposure to sunlight can be tolerated. Individuals with light skin and hair do not tolerate sunlight well because they do not tan to provide protection from and tolerance to sunlight. The repeated exposure of an individual with little natural pigment of the skin to sunlight conditions his skin to the development of skin cancer later in life. The majority of skin cancers on the surface of the body exposed to sunlight occurs in those individuals who have little natural tolerance to sunlight. (See Etiology of Neoplasia, Chapter 5, p. 112.)

X-ray radiation is another form of radiant energy which produces cell damage. This type of radiation is much more potent than ultraviolet rays. Mild application such as is used for diagnostic x rays is

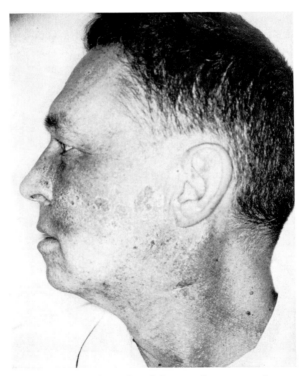

Figure 7. Acute changes in skin of mid-face and upper neck caused by cobalt irradiation. The skin is darker in color, dry and scaly; hair is absent.

of little significance, but larger quantities, either in a single exposure or in repeated small exposures, result in tissue injury. The initial changes due to significant x-ray irradiation include redness and slight swelling of the skin and loss of hair. These changes subside gradually if the irradiation has not been too intense. However, if the radiation is intense, cells are destroyed and an open sore frequently occurs called an x-ray burn. If the dose of x ray is intense but short causing tissue death, the acute tissue changes subside, but permanent injury to blood vessels and tissue is evident (Fig. 7). The skin of the area is thin, slightly scarred, devoid of hair, and the superficial blood vessels are dilated and tortuous. The pale, scarred skin has delicate, red spider-web markings produced by the tortuous vessels (Fig. 8). If bone is irradiated, similar changes are present in its blood vessels and the metabolism and healing power of the bone is decreased. If such irradiated bone is subsequently subjected to injury or infection, necrosis occurs owing to the poor circulation. The necrotic bone is separated and expelled from the area (sequestration). Irradiation also results in rampant caries (Fig. 9).

Small doses of x-ray irradiation over long periods condition the skin to the development of cancer. Various parts of the body are more severely affected by irradiation than others. The gonads are very susceptible to x ray and exposure may produce sterility. Bone

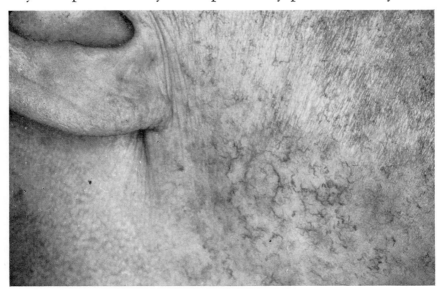

Figure 8. *Chronic effects of irradiation.* In front of the ear the skin is atrophic and finely wrinkled. Below the ear it is smooth and depigmented. There is a "spider-web" effect produced by tortuous dilated vessels (telangiectasia).

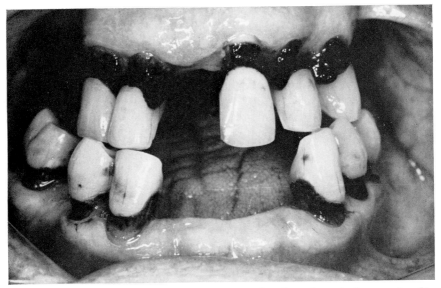

Figure 9. Extensive cervical caries often result when there is intense irradiation of the oral region.

marrow is also very sensitive to x-ray irradiation; and if there is total body exposure, the bone marrow may be destroyed. When the bone marrow is destroyed, the body is unable to cope with infection and death results. Irradiation from other sources of radiant energy, such as radium and radioactive materials, produces a similar type of injury.

Electrical energy causes damage to tissue. The severity of the damage depends upon the intensity of the current and the electrical resistance of the tissue. When a sufficiently high current passes through the body, death results because of paralysis of the respiratory center.

Microorganisms

An invasion of the body by microorganisms can produce injury locally and systemically. Bacteria may produce toxins which are transported to areas distant from their site of entry and thus cause systemic disease. Bacteria may be transported by the blood stream (bacteremia) to sites distant from their portal of entry to produce tissue damage. Transient bacteremia, resulting from the extraction or scaling of teeth, is a significant cause of subacute bacterial endocarditis. In this instance, bacteria, most often Streptococcus viridans, gain entrance to the blood stream and lodge in damaged heart valves where they produce endocarditis. The damaged heart may be congenital in origin or acquired, as from rheumatic fever. It is for this reason that patients with a history of rheumatic fever and congenital heart disease require careful evaluation and antibiotic medication prior to scaling or extraction procedures.

The cellular reaction to microorganisms is called infection. Each type of organism incites a different reaction either of the entire organism or of a particular part; therefore the reaction is designated a specific disease. Infection is discussed in more detail in Chapter 4, page 67.

Psychologic Causes

When individuals are subjected to severe psychologic conflicts or tensions, they may be unable to resolve their conflicts and develop abnormal patterns of behavior as a means of escape from reality. These individuals have mental disease. This is a very important and common form of disease in our present-day society. When an individual is under severe emotional strain, the stress may affect various parts of the body, especially the endocrine glands, and cause them to function abnormally. This results in various forms of tissue alterations. Such diseases have psychosomatic factors as a cause. Peptic ulcer is a good example of a psychosomatic disease.

DEVELOPMENTAL FACTORS

Disease may result from a disturbance in the development of a tissue or a part of the body. If some cells of a developing tissue are injured, further development may be limited, resulting in an abnormal or defective tissue. The defect may be large in magnitude and incompatible with life, or it may be minor and of little consequence as far as function of the organism is concerned. Such developmental defects are designated anomalies. If present at birth they are called congenital anomalies. A developmental anomaly is usually the result of an alteration in anatomic form, but disturbances in function, such as failure of an organ to carry out metabolism of a particular substance, may also occur.

Hereditary and developmental disease processes may be easily confused. The presence of a disease at birth does not necessarily indicate it as hereditary in origin, for many developmental disturbances also are present at birth. Improper development of a tissue may occur some time after birth and be a late manifestation of a developmental disturbance. Developmental anomalies sometimes manifested at birth must be differentiated from disease processes occurring after the complete development of a tissue or part of the body.

It is possible for environmental factors to cause profound defects at any time during the development of the embryo or fetus. Teratogenic agents include certain drugs, irradiation, some viruses, and at least one parasite. The term *teratology* refers to the study or science of malformations and monstrosities, and the term *teratogenic* to the capability of causing malformations and monsters. Probably the most widely publicized teratogenic syndrome has been the thalidomide effect on the development of the limbs, especially the upper extremities. The defect, *phocomelia,* is characterized by an absence of or presence of imperfectly formed forearms, thighs, and legs. Maternal infection with rubella (German measles) during the early months of pregnancy may cause developmental defects involving the heart, brain, ears, and eyes. The salivary gland virus usually produces only a mild reaction to a mother during pregnancy, but the infection may produce widespread damage in utero to the developing fetus. Irradiation of the human fetus may result in a variety of defects, often the same as those considered to be due to genetic change. Such defects caused by irradiation include mongolism, microcephaly (small head), retinoblastoma (tumor of the retina), facial deformities, and many other defects of the eyes, brain, and skeleton.

Cleft lip and palate are developmental disturbances occurring in utero during development of these parts and are present at birth. Because they are manifest at birth, they are congenital defects. Epithelial inclusions in a branchial cleft occur early in the development of the face and neck, but the development of cysts from the included epithelium to form branchial cleft cysts may not be evident until adult life. Such a cyst is developmental but not congenital since it was not evident at birth. Dentigerous cysts are disturbances in the development of the tooth germ which are initiated after birth and appear later in the life of an individual. Anomalous development of the valves or septae of the heart results in abnormal structure and function of the organ. The "blue baby" is an example of this variety of congenital anomaly.

Disease processes of various types may be hereditary in origin and be manifested at birth or may appear later in the life of the individual. Hereditary diseases may be alterations in form or function. Although the individual does not have a disease process as the result of hereditary factors, he may develop a constitutional background which predisposes him to the development of certain diseases. Thus heredity plays an important part in the development of disease.

Developmental disturbances of some slight degree are present in a large part of the population; more severe disturbances are present in fewer individuals. Even though few in number, developmental disturbances make up an important segment of disease.

SUMMARY

The largest category of disease is provided by numerous extrinsic factors which are continuously active in the environment. Extrinsic factors are increasing in importance and number owing to our industrial advancement and the use of atomic energy. The continually changing pattern is due to the elimination or control of some disease factors and the development of new factors which cause disease. The pattern of disease changes with each generation. Heart disease, which 40 years ago was rated fourth or fifth as a cause of death, is now first. This shift in the position of heart disease as a cause of death is the result of the control of some diseases, such as smallpox, pneumonia, and typhoid fever, which, in the past, frequently caused death, and the conditions of tension under which we now live in our highly mechanistic society which predisposes to heart disease. Patterns of disease are continually changing as the result of elimination or control of some of the older factors responsible for disease and the rise of new etiologic factors.

BIBLIOGRAPHY

Brukner, R. J., Rickles, N. H., and Porter, D. R.: Hypophosphatasia with premature shedding of teeth and aplasia of cementum. Oral Surg., 15:1351, 1962.

Carvel, R. I.: Palmo-plantar hyperkeratosis and premature periodontal destruction. J. Oral Med., 24:73, 1969.

Falconer, D. S.: The inheritance of liability to certain diseases estimated from the incidence among relatives. Ann. Hum. Genet., 29:51, 1965.

German, J.: Studying human chromosomes today. Amer. Sci., 58:182, 1970.

Gorlin, R.: Genetic disorders affecting mucous membranes. Oral Surg., 28:512, 1969.

Gorlin, R. J., Stallard, R. E., and Shapiro, B. L.: Genetics and periodontal disease. J. Periodont., 38:5, 1967.

Medical Research Council: The hazards to man of nuclear and allied radiations. London, Her Majesty's Stationary Office, 1960.

Naeye, R. L., and Blane, W.: Pathogenesis of congenital rubella. J.A.M.A., 194:1277, 1965.

Neel, J. V., and Schull, W. J.: Studies on the potential genetic effects of the atomic bombs. Acta Genet. (Basel), 6:183, 1956.

Ochoa, S.: The chemical basis of heredity—the genetic code. Bull. N.Y. Acad. Med., 40:387, 1964.

Poyton, H. G.: The effects of irradiation on teeth. Oral Surg., 26:639, 1968.

Taussig, H. B.: The thalidomide syndrome. Sci. Amer., 207:29, 1962.

Valentine, G. H.: The Chromosome Disorders, An Introduction for Clinicians. London, Heineman, 1966.

World Health Organization: Radiation hazards in perspective. Technical Report Series, No. 248, Geneva, 1962.

Chapter 3

DEVELOPMENTAL DISTURBANCES

The development of the body starts at the time of the union of the male and female sex cells and the pooling of their nuclei in the process of fertilization. In effect, the fertilized egg cell is a new cell produced by the two sex cells. Following union, the fertilized egg cell undergoes a series of cell divisions and multiplication to begin the development of a new individual. As the cells multiply they also undergo differentiation so that they assume the characteristics of various tissues of the body. The formation of an organism as complex as the human body by such a process of proliferation and differentiation of cells provides many possibilities for error. When one group of cells fails to grow or differentiate, another group dependent on them for development may be affected. This entire chain of events may be inhibited because of changes in a few cells. The results of disturbances in the orderly sequence of events in the development of the individual are called developmental defects, or anomalies.

Because of the complex nature of the process of development of the body, unlimited possibilities for disturbances in development are present; these disturbances constitute important manifestations of disease. The face is a common location for developmental disturbances owing to its complex pattern of growth, and therefore a brief review of the embryology of the face and jaws will precede a discussion of the more common and important developmental disturbances of these areas.

EMBRYOLOGY OF THE FACE

The development of the facial region is a complex process of selective growth (proliferation) of parts which, as they grow, undergo changes in cellular detail (differentiation) to form the various structures of the face. The differentiation of the cells responsible for the formation of a part may depend upon some change in other cells of the immediate area. This process is called dependent differ-

4

entiation, and it plays an important part in the development of the face. As the cells of the body proliferate they have the capacity to follow a particular pattern of growth to form a structure of specific architecture. This process is called morphodifferentiation and is evident in the formation of the face and oral structures.

The head region of the embryo starts its development at about the fourth week of embryonic life by the development of a rounded prominence (the forebrain) on the cephalic (head) end of the embryo. This prominence folds forward and downward (ventral and inferior) to form a groove (the oral groove) representing the rudimentary oral cavity. The lower boundary of the groove is the first branchial bar. Lateral boundaries of the groove develop by proliferation of cells from the sides and top (lateral and superior) portions of the first branchial bar.

The first branchial bar forms the lower jaw (mandible) (Fig. 10A, B) and the portions that develop laterally grow forward to form part of the upper jaw (maxilla) and the roof of the mouth (palate). While these lateral processes are developing, there is an outgrowth in the center of the forebrain which grows downward between the two lateral processes of the developing maxilla (Fig. 10C, D). This outgrowth forms the middle part of the upper face and is called the median process. This process develops two lateral

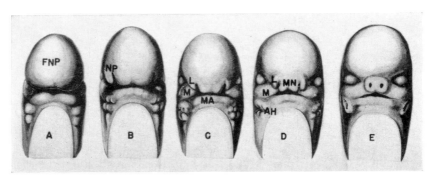

Figure 10. *Development of the face.* A, Formation of stomadeum by anterior folding of the forebrain with development of frontal nasal process (FNP). Folds below rudimentary oral cavity are branchial bars. B, Development of globular processes from frontal nasal process and development of lateral nasal process (NP). C, Development of maxillary process (M) from superior portion of first branchial bar and nearly completed mandible (MA) from inferior portion of first branchial bar. D, More complete development of frontal nasal process to show medial and nasal process (MN) below which are the paired globular processes. Lateral nasal process (L), maxilla (M), and auricular hillock (AH). E, Nearly complete development of the face. (Courtesy of Dr. James K. Avery.)

pits which separate the median process into two lateral processes and one medial process. They are the lateral nasal processes and the medial nasal process.

As the lateral nasal processes develop, they push the olfactory pits toward the midline and compress the medial nasal process to a thin strip. The lateral nasal processes form the sides of the nose, and the median process forms the center of the nose. The inferior portion of the median nasal process proliferates as a globular mass of tissue (the globular process) to form the upper midportion of the maxilla (the portion containing the central and lateral incisors). While the median nasal and lateral nasal processes are developing, the maxillary process grows forward to meet the globular process. When all the structures have developed and come in contact, they fuse to form the completed face. The face thus develops from several individual parts fusing together to form the final structure (Fig. 10E). The two lateral halves of the maxillary process meet in the midline to form the posterior part of the palate. They fuse with the globular process to form the anterior palate. The opening of the oral cavity is produced by the incomplete fusion of the mandibular and maxillary processes of the face.

In a process as complex as the development of the face, there are many possibilities for some failure of formation to occur. Some of these occur quite frequently, whereas others are rare. The more common and most significant ones will be discussed in some detail.

DISTURBANCES OF THE UPPER FACE

Clefts

A cleft is one of the most frequently occurring disturbances resulting from the failure of fusion of the various processes from which the face develops. Any defect that results from failure of fusion of any of the facial processes is called a cleft. The most common clefts occur in the region of the upper lip and palate (Fig. 11). Clefts rarely occur in the lower jaw. Failure of the maxillary process to fuse with the globular process may result in a cleft on one or both sides of the midline. When the cleft is on one side of the midline, it is unilateral; when it occurs on both sides, it is bilateral. This type of cleft simulates the upper lip of the rabbit and thus is designated harelip. Such failure of fusion may involve only a portion of the lip or all of the lip. When all of the lip is involved, it may extend into the jaw and palate. Any combination and extent of cleft of the lip and palate may occur. In some instances only the two lateral portions of the maxillary process which form the palate may fail to unite and a cleft of the palate alone results.

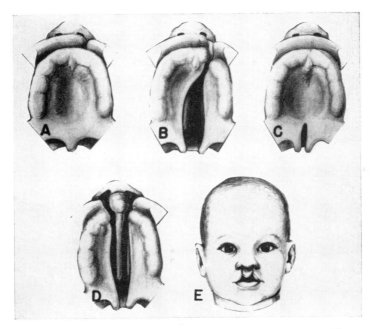

Figure 11. *Hare lip and cleft palate.* A, Cleft lip only; B, cleft of lip, jaw, and palate; C, incomplete cleft of palate, bifid uvula; D, bilateral cleft of lip and jaw, extensive midline cleft of palate; E, front view of bilateral cleft.

Reports of the prevalence of clefts of the lip and palate indicate that some variation in their frequency occurs according to geographic regions and race. The frequency of occurrence is reported to be one out of 954 births in Holland (Sanders) and one out of 1200 births in the United States (Lyons). Racial variation of cleft of the palate and lips is not readily explained, but is probably related to the various causes of disturbances in development. The etiology of cleft lip (harelip) and cleft palate has not been definitely established, but it appears that heredity plays an important part; however, such factors as nutrition, mechanical interference during development, and specific diseases may be contributing factors. Cleft palate is frequently associated with other types of developmental disturbances.

Infants born with harelip and cleft palate are usually able to live, but present many problems in care and treatment. Infants with clefts are unable to suckle well and present feeding problems; they have a tendency to aspirate food and therefore are susceptible to respiratory disease. Older children have problems of speech and esthetics as well as social and psychologic problems. To prevent the development of these problems during childhood and yet not interfere with growth centers, it is desirable to treat such individuals at an early age. Clefts of the lip usually are treated by surgical closure in the first few months of life, and cleft of the palate at about 18 months of age. In some instances, surgery is only partially successful and the clefts must be treated by prosthetic appliances and orthodontic procedures. Today, in most large medical centers and in some states, special cleft palate clinics are staffed with teams of surgeons, dentists, speech therapists, psychologists, and social workers to treat patients with clefts of the lip and palate.

Fissural Defects

In addition to the development of clefts from the failure of facial processes to fuse, less severe disturbances may occur in the lines of fusion. Facial processes are covered by epithelium which is obliterated at the time of fusion of the processes. In some instances, fusion may be complete, except for the persistence of epithelium in a small area of the line of fusion. Many variations of persistent epithelium occur. The epithelium may persist in a localized area through the full thickness of the line of fusion to produce an epithelial-lined tract from the outer to the inner surface of the fused processes. An epithelial-lined tube or tract open at both ends is called a fistula. The persistent epithelium may have continuity with only one surface to form a blind tract or tube with only one opening on one of the surfaces of the fused processes. This tract of residual epithelium with a blind end is called a *sinus*. When the persistent or residual epithelium forms a closed space in a line of fusion, the defect is called a *fissural cyst*.

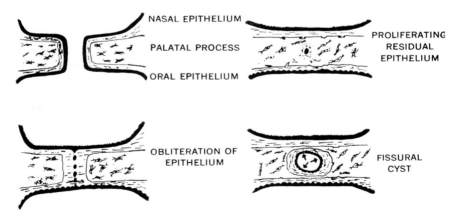

Figure 12. Formation of fissural cyst in palate.

CYSTS. Examples of fissural defects may be seen in various areas of the face and mouth. Cysts are by far the most common of the fissural defects and occur in the midline of the palate (midpalatine cyst) (Figs. 12, 13), in the line of fusion between the maxillary and globular processes (globulomaxillary cyst), or in the area of fusion between the two lateral portions of the palate and the medial nasal process (nasopalatine cyst) (Fig. 14). Fissural cysts may appear in front of the ear (preauricular cyst) owing to the persistence of epithelium between the superior and inferior halves of the first branchial bar. Sinuses occurring in this region are called preauric-

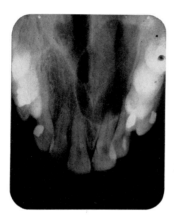

Figure 13. *Fissural cyst of palate*. Cyst originates in midline but extends laterally as it meets floor of nose and maxillary sinus.

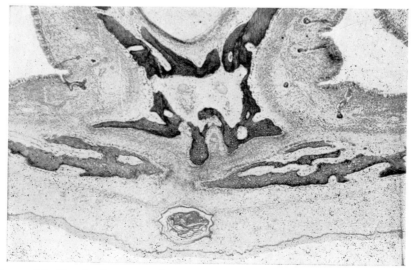

Figure 14. Developing nasopalatine cyst beneath palatal mucosa at floor of nose. Nasal cavities can be seen at upper right and left of figure.

ular sinuses and may be present bilaterally. Cysts also occur owing to the persistence of epithelium between the other branchial bars (branchial cysts) and are present beneath the angle of the jaw on the lateral surface of the neck. A cyst slowly increases in size due to an accumulation of tissue fluid within the cystic space, and thus produces a swelling and deformity necessitating treatment by surgical excision. If the removal is complete and all of the epithelial lining is removed, the condition is eliminated and there is no recurrence. However, if some of the lining is not removed, the cyst may re-form.

Other inclusions, usually some element of the skin, may occur in fusion lines. Sebaceous glands are frequently included in the line of fusion between the maxillary and mandibular processes. Such ectopic sebaceous glands (Fordyce's spots) are found just beneath the buccal mucosa along the line of occlusion of the teeth. They may present opposite the last molar, around the parotid papillae, sometimes near the angle of the mouth and occasionally on the gingiva; they usually occur bilaterally. These glands appear in the mucosa singularly or in groups as small (1 to 2 millimeters), slightly elevated chamois-colored spots (Fig. 15). When the inclusions are numerous and close together, they produce a yellowish, rough plaque. These glandular inclusions may be seen on the exposed vermilion border of the lip as extensions from the skin beneath the lip mucosa. About 80 percent of the adult population have these inclusions. Fordyce's spots are of no serious significance as far as the health of the patient is concerned, but may cause the patient to be alarmed when first noticed. They are not seen in children before puberty, inasmuch as sebaceous glands are a part of the secondary sex characteristics activated during puberty by hormonal stimulation from the gonads. Although no treatment is indicated,

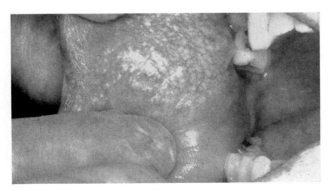

Figure 15. Fordyce's spots in buccal mucosa.

patients should be assured of the innocuous nature of Fordyce's spots.

DEVELOPMENTAL CYSTS.   Developmental cysts may occur in association with the salivary glands, especially those located in the floor of the mouth (submaxillary and sublingual glands), and the submucosal glands (accessory salivary glands) of the lips, buccal mucosa, and palate. During the development of a major salivary gland, its ductal system may not develop completely so that some of the ducts within the gland do not establish communication with an excretory duct but end in the tissue as a blind tube. Because of the absence of an opening for excretion of the saliva, the secretions, chiefly mucin, accumulate in the duct. The accumulation of salivary secretions causes the duct to distend, which results in a space lined by ductal epithelium and filled with secretion. When this condition occurs in association with the major salivary glands, the distended epithelial-lined spaces filled with mucinous secretions are called *mucous retention cysts* (Fig. 90); those arising from the same condition in the accessory glands are called *mucoceles* (Figs. 16, 88). Frequently the mucinous material escapes from the distended ducts into the surrounding tissues. In some instances, a mucous retention cyst or mucocele may be *acquired* owing to the plugging of a duct by a stone (sialolith) or by scar tissue following an injury. When

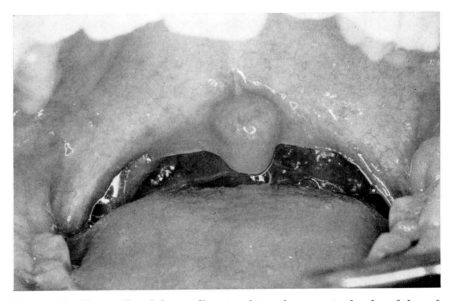

Figure 16. The small nodular swelling involving the posterior border of the soft palate and the uvula is due to obstruction of mucous gland ducts with retention of secretion.

the accumulation of mucin increases in ducts or tissues which are in close proximity to the surface of the mucosa, a visible swelling is produced. The accumulated mucin can be seen through the thin mucosa and imparts a blister-like appearance to the lesion. These cysts frequently rupture owing to pressure and injury allowing fluid to escape into the tissue or the mouth. The ruptured area heals but the fluid accumulates again to produce a new swelling. These cysts are eliminated by surgical removal.

DISTURBANCES OF THE TONGUE

The tongue develops from the posterior and lateral internal surfaces of the first, second, and third branchial bars as three nodular swellings. The middle nodule, arising from the posterior area, develops into the base of the tongue, whereas the two lateral nodules develop into the body of the tongue. In the early stages of development of the tongue, the growth of the medial portion is much more advanced than the lateral portions; however, as development progresses the lateral portions usually outgrow the medial portion so that the medial portion is not evident in the mature tongue. In less than 1 percent of the population, a part of the outline of the medial portion persists as a smooth, elevated, mamelonated, rounded or flat, rhomboid zone in the midline of the posterior part of the tongue just anterior to the circumvallate papillae. This abnormality is called *median rhomboid glossitis* (Fig. 17). Rarely the two lateral portions of the tongue do not completely fuse resulting in a notched or forked tongue. This is manifest as an irregular V-shaped notch in the tip of the tongue called *bifid tongue*.

The anterior one-third of the tongue is usually free or partially attached to the floor of the mouth by a thin strip of tissue extending from the midline of the ventral surface of the tongue to the floor

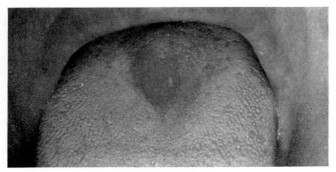

Figure 17. *Median rhomboid glossitis*. Smooth rhomboidal elevation without papillae on the posterior one-third of dorsum of tongue.

of the mouth (lingual frenum). In some instances the frenum is short and attached too near the tip of the tongue so that the tongue is bound tightly to the floor of the mouth preventing normal mobility (Fig. 18). This abnormality, *tongue tie* or *ankyloglossia,* sometimes causes difficulty in suckling, eating, or speaking. In such cases it is necessary to clip the frenum to permit the tongue to move freely.

Normally the tongue is smooth in its contour and is covered by fine projections, papillae, which give it a slightly shaggy appearance. Food and cell debris entrapped in these fine hair-like papillae produce a somewhat velvet-like appearance to the tongue designated the "coat of the tongue." The coating of the tongue varies in color and amount depending upon the abundance of saliva and the texture and the color of foods eaten. The coat is usually grayish-yellow but may be brown from coffee, tea, or smoking; red from colored candy; green from chlorophyl lozenges or certain toothpastes; or other colors depending upon the substance taken into the mouth. A "coated tongue" is generally of little dental or medical significance except as it relates to oral hygiene. In fact, the absence of coating may be of significance in anemias and vitamin deficiencies.

So-called *hairy tongue* is perhaps only an exaggerated form of coated tongue, but the retained filiform papillae are longer and are localized to a limited area of the tongue (Fig. 19). The retained filiform papillae are like hair in both texture and color, usually being dark-brown or black in color and a few millimeters to a centimeter in length. When the papillae are long, the patient may feel their presence, but usually they are discovered by observation. The retention of the papillae is enhanced by the use of hydrogen peroxide as a mouthwash, use of antibiotics, presence of yeast in large

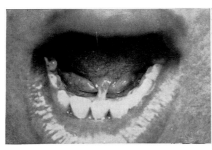 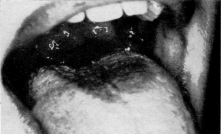

Figure 18. *Ankyloglossia.* Attachment of lingual frenum from tip of tongue to lingual aspect of gingiva.

Figure 19. *Black hairy tongue.* Accentuated filiform papillae on posterior one-third of the dorsum of tongue simulate coarse hairs.

numbers in the oral flora, and in some instances there is no identifiable cause.

Furrowed tongue is an abnormality of the tongue present in about 25 percent of the population in which the dorsum of the tongue develops heavy folds (Fig. 20). The folds may follow a regular geometric pattern or they may be irregular, without pattern. The entire dorsum of the tongue is involved, and the deep furrows between the folds may extend onto the lateral borders. The depth of the furrows may not be readily discernible until the tongue is extended or mildly stretched. Geographic tongue is superimposed upon furrowed tongue in many instances. Irritation in the furrows has been suggested as a possible cause of geographic tongue. Some writers believe that furrowed tongue is congenital, whereas others think that it is acquired. In favor of its being acquired is the fact that it rarely occurs in children.

Another anomaly of the tongue present in about 5 percent of the population is *geographic tongue* also designated wandering rash or glossitis migrans (Fig. 21). This condition is frequently associated with furrowed tongue, but may be seen on a smooth tongue. When associated with furrowed tongue, the change usually starts as a loss of filiform papillae about a fissure. The loss of papillae extends from the fissure in a widening arc and the zone of separation from the normal surface of the tongue appears as a white line. When the papillae are completely lost, the epithelium is thin and the under-lying tissue is near enough to the surface of the tongue to be seen readily and to give the narrow area involved a reddish appearance. The epithelium then regenerates and new papillae start to form; this process produces a smooth, slightly purplish zone. The process of

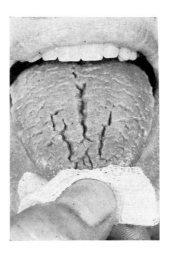

Figure 20. *Furrowed tongue.*

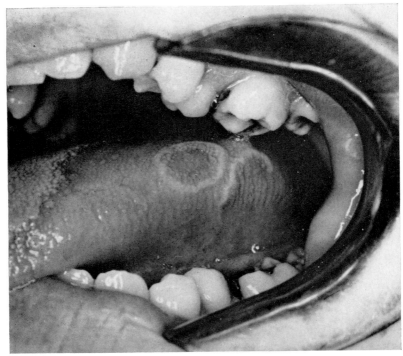

Figure 21. *Geographic tongue.* There are two active lesions on the lateral
border indicated by the white circular and arcuate boundaries. The
lesions are superimposed on a larger area of previous desquamative
activity.

depapillation, thinning of the epithelium and its regeneration, extends progressively outward from a fissure for a variable distance
and then ceases, only to start again in the same or another area.
Because some lesions are healing while new ones are starting, there
usually are several areas of variable size and shape which present a
continually changing picture to the tongue so it appears different
each time it is observed. The pattern of involvement is suggestive
of a map and for this reason it has been designated geographic
tongue. Geographic tongue occurs in children as well as adults and
may be present for a lifetime. It rarely produces symptoms and the
patient usually only becomes aware of it through observation. In a
few cases a smarting or burning sensation may be present, especially
when eating highly seasoned or hot foods. The cause of this condition is believed to be associated with the action of bacteria in the
coat of the tongue or in the fissures of furrowed tongue where food
debris or organisms are trapped and produce irritation. This condi-

tion is of little or no significance to the individual and treatment is not indicated. When treatment is attempted, it usually is unsuccessful.

DISTURBANCES OF THE JAWS

The most common disturbance in the development of the jaws is the cleft of the jaw and palate discussed under clefts of the face. Other disturbances in the jaws are associated with alterations of growth due to injuries to the jaws at birth as the result of forceps deliveries or to infections of the ear and about the jaws. Injury or infection in the region of the condyle may prevent growth, which results in a lack of development of the mandible (micrognathia). In this case the individual has a receding chin (Fig. 22) or appears to have no chin (Andy Gump physiognomy). There may be unequal growth of the two sides of the jaws resulting in an asymmetry of the face. Overgrowth of the mandible or lack of development of the maxilla results in a protrusion of the mandible giving a pugnacious

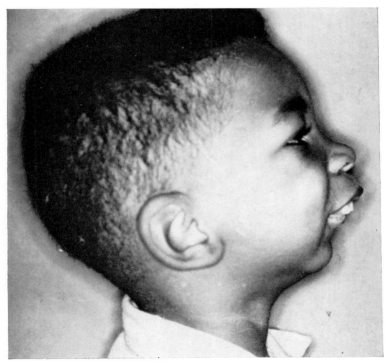

Figure 22. *Micrognathia.* This facial disturbance began early in life as indicated by marked discrepancy in development of mandible compared to maxilla.

appearance to the individual. The jaws may fail to develop sufficiently to provide adequate space for accommodation of the teeth resulting in an irregularly formed arch and crowding of the teeth. Unequal development of the jaws also prevents the jaws from coming together properly, which results in malocclusion. Crowded teeth in poor occlusion are functionally and esthetically undesirable. Because malocclusion detracts considerably from the appearance of the individual, psychologic problems may arise and affect the personality of the individual. Deformities of position and arrangement of teeth may be corrected by orthodontic procedures thereby improving the esthetics and thus the psychologic outlook of the patient.

EMBRYOLOGY OF THE TEETH

About the sixth week of embryonic life the development of the teeth starts as a proliferation of the cells on the crest of the rudimentary jaw (Fig. 23). This selectively localized growth of cells on the crest of the ridge produces a strand of epithelium called the dental lamina. At about the tenth week, certain areas of the dental lamina proliferate more rapidly than others and bud-like swellings are produced. Each of these bud-like masses of epithelium represents the beginning of the formation of an individual tooth and is termed the tooth bud.

Cells in different areas of the tooth bud proliferate at different rates making some of the cells of the dental lamina appear as if they

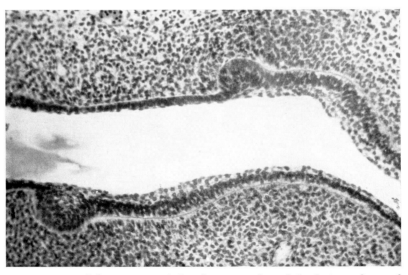

Figure 23. *Dental lamina.* Initial development of tooth buds in embryo of six weeks.

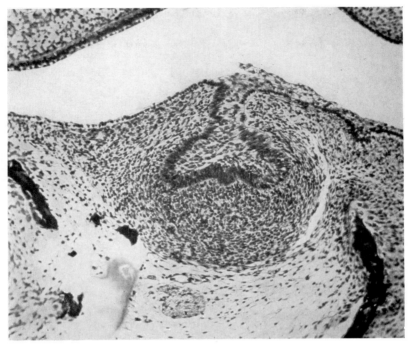

Figure 24. *Cap stage of tooth bud.* Note concentration of mesenchymal cells around tooth bud indicating initial formation of dental sac and dental papillae. Black areas at right and left are developing bony crypt.

are growing into or invaginating the surrounding tissues. In effect, the process of differential growth rate results in the formation of a cap-like appearance of the developing tooth bud (cap stage) (Figs. 24, 25). Further growth and selective proliferation of the peripheral cells change the appearance of the tooth bud to a bell-like structure (bell stage) (Fig. 26). This process of selective growth of cells to provide a characteristic shape to a structure is morphodifferentiation. The process of proliferation and morphodifferentiation of the epithelium also influences the proliferation of mesenchymal tissue in contact with the inner aspect of the epithelium of the bell-like tooth bud. This area of mesenchymal tissue within the bell-like arrangement of the epithelium is the dental papilla (Fig. 26). The epithelium arranged in the bell-like fashion is designated the enamel organ. The enamel organ and the dental papilla constitute the tooth germ. The enamel organ is now divided into distinct layers with the cells of each layer having a characteristic pattern; the epithelium forming the outer surface of the bell-like tooth bud is the *outer enamel*

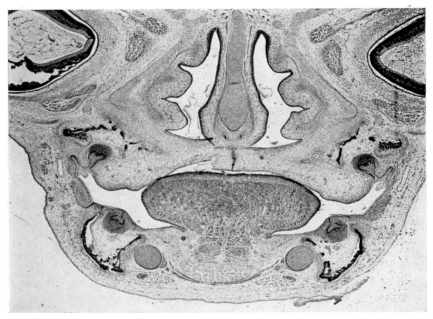

Figure 25. Frontal section through face of embryo of seven weeks. Note relation of tooth germ to oral cavity; early development of mucobuccal fold lateral to the dental lamina; outline of developing mandible.

epithelium, and the epithelium forming the inner aspect of the bell-like structure is the *inner enamel epithelium* (Fig. 26).

As the tooth germ increases in size, cells of the inner enamel epithelium change in shape and become columnar. Cells of the outer enamel epithelium retain their original shape, while cells between the inner and outer enamel epithelium increase in number and develop a stellate character. This change in shape and accompanying proliferation is histodifferentiation. As the inner enamel epithelium develops, its cells differentiate into two layers: the inner-most layer composed of a single row of tall columnar cells (the ameloblasts), and an outer layer of polyhedral cells four to six cells in thickness (the stratum intermedium). The outer-most layer of the enamel organ retains the character of squamous epithelium. Between the outer and inner enamel epithelium the cells become stellate with numerous long intercellular processes producing a mesh-like pattern (the stellate reticulum). As proliferation progresses, morphodifferentiation continues and the configuration of a particular tooth becomes evident. One enamel organ develops the configuration of an incisor, another a cuspid, and another a molar. At the same time histodifferentiation continues in both the ameloblastic layer of the

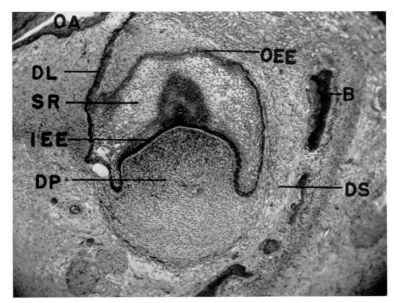

Figure 26. *Bell stage of developing tooth.* Oral cavity (OA), dental lamina (DL), outer enamel epithelium (OEE), stellate reticulum (SR), inner enamel epithelium (IEE), dental papillae (DP), dental sac (DS), bone (B) of developing jaw.

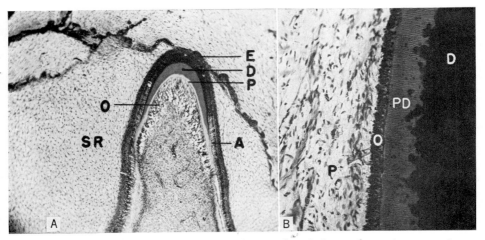

Figure 27. *Dentin formation.* A, Initial enamel and dentin formation over tip of cusp; dentin (D), predentin (P), odontoblasts (O), enamel matrix (E), ameloblasts (A), stellate reticulum (SR). B, Later stage of dentin formation; odontoblasts (O), predentin with dark spherical areas of calcification (PD), calcified dentin (D), dental pulp (P).

enamel organ and the dental papilla. The ameloblasts become tall
and are arranged parallel to each other and perpendicular to the
border of the dental papilla. The basement membrane of the ameloblasts in contact with the dental papilla thickens and is designated
the dento-enamel membrane, which is the landmark for the future
dento-enamel junction.

The formation of the dento-enamel membrane influences the peripheral cells of the dental papilla to differentiate into columnar cells
oriented perpendicularly to the enamel membrane. These cells are
the odontoblasts, responsible for the formation of dentin (Fig. 27).
After the odontoblasts differentiate and start to form dentin, the
ameloblasts become functional and produce enamel. Each amelo-
blast forms an individual enamel rod as it moves away from the
dento-enamel junction toward the outer enamel epithelium. The
movement of the ameloblasts toward the outer enamel epithelium
compresses the stellate reticulum causing it to undergo atrophy
(Fig. 28). When the full thickness of the enamel is completed, the
ameloblasts of the inner enamel epithelium atrophy, revert to
squamous cells, and unite with the outer enamel epithelium. The
completed enamel of the crown of the tooth is now covered by a
single layer of squamous epithelium (the reduced enamel epithelium). The reduced enamel epithelium remains on the surface of
the tooth as it erupts into the oral cavity.

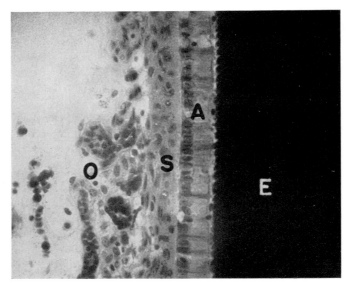

Figure 28. *Formation of enamel.* Enamel (E), ameloblasts (A), stratum intermedium (S), outer enamel epithelium (O) about capillaries.

While the enamel is being formed, the odontoblasts form dentin as they move inward from the dento-enamel junction. As dentin is formed it surrounds the dental papilla now designated the dental pulp. The process of dentin formation becomes slower when dentin reaches its normal size, but continues as long as the pulp is vital.

During the time the enamel organ is undergoing proliferation, morphodifferentiation, and histodifferentiation, the connective tissue surrounding it proliferates and differentiates into the dental sac, responsible for the formation of the supporting mechanism of the teeth, i.e., the cementum, the periodontal membrane, and the alveolar bone.

Also during the period the teeth are developing, they are surrounded by the bone of the developing jaws. The cavity within the bone in which the tooth is being formed is the dental crypt. The first teeth formed from the dental lamina are the deciduous or primary teeth. After the deciduous teeth are partially formed the dental lamina sends off secondary buds, which develop in the same manner but more slowly than primary teeth to form the permanent or succedaneous teeth (Fig. 29).

All permanent teeth are called succedaneous except the molars. The dental lamina proliferates posteriorly to form the tooth buds of the permanent molars (Fig. 29). All of the enamel organs do not develop at the same rate of speed, thus some teeth are completed before others are formed. The result is different times of eruption for various groups of teeth. Groups of teeth develop at specific rates so that the times of eruption follow a definite chronologic order and their appearance in the mouth can be anticipated at specific ages.

Because of the complex nature of odontogenesis wherein cells undergo morphodifferentiation and histodifferentiation and where the changes in one group of cells are dependent upon another group of cells, there are many possibilities for disturbances in the development of the teeth. These disturbances may be in the formation or eruption of one or of all the teeth.

DISTURBANCES OF THE TEETH

Developmental disturbances of the teeth may be manifest by variations in number, position, size, shape, eruption, or structure. Such disturbances may occur in association with some more generalized disorder or may occur independently. Some of the more common developmental anomalies will be discussed.

Disturbances in the *number* of teeth may occur when all or some of the teeth fail to develop (agenesis or anodontia) or because too many teeth develop (hyperodontia or supernumerary teeth). Agenesis may occur with any disturbance of ectodermal tissue which

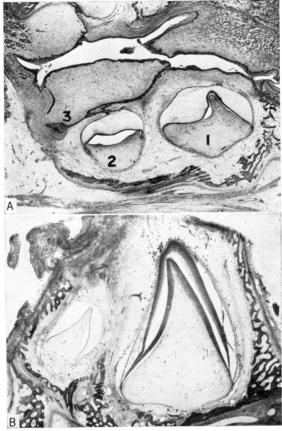

Figure 29. *Enamel organ.* A, (1) Beginning dentin formation at tip of cusp
of first deciduous molar; (2) advanced bell stage of second deciduous molar; (3) posterior proliferation of dental lamina with initiation of tooth bud for first permanent molar. B, Partial development
of enamel and dentin of crown of deciduous incisor, and development of enamel organ of succedaneous incisor.

prevents its proliferation and differentiation into highly specialized
cells (ectodermal dysplasia). In such instances, all or some of the
teeth may fail to develop. This disturbance is associated with anhidrotic ectodermal dysplasia manifested by a failure to develop the
specialized skin appendages such as sweat glands, hair follicles, and
nails. In other instances, a single tooth or type of tooth may fail to
develop. This type of anodontia usually is hereditary and both
parent and offspring may have the same teeth absent. The third
molars, maxillary lateral incisors, and the first bicuspids are the most
frequently congenitally absent teeth in the order named.

In some hereditary diseases an individual may develop more than the normal number of teeth. The extra, or supernumerary, teeth are most often the maxillary incisors or molars. Supernumerary teeth are usually abnormal in size and shape and may or may not erupt. If eruption occurs it is usually associated with abnormal position (Fig. 30A, B, C). They may fail to erupt and prevent the eruption of adjacent normal teeth. From time to time patients report they know of someone with a third dentition; however, no authenticated case of a third dentition has been reported. Occasionally babies born with teeth have also been reported. Usually they are not true teeth but are tooth-like structures formed from the mucosa over the area from which the dental lamina is initiated. Such "teeth" may be shed quickly or may have to be removed. They represent overzealous proliferation of oral epithelium in the region of the dental lamina.

Disturbances in eruption may be manifest as precocious or delayed eruption. The deciduous teeth may erupt earlier than normal, usually followed by early shedding of deciduous teeth and early eruption of the permanent dentition. Early eruption of teeth may be due to hyperfunction of the pituitary or thyroid glands.

Delayed eruption of teeth may involve all or part of the dentition. The entire deciduous dentition may be delayed as well as a corresponding delay in the eruption of the permanent dentition and is usually associated with delay in the general growth of the individual. Individual teeth may be delayed in eruption because they develop in an abnormal position and impinge against adjacent teeth. This is especially true of third molars and occasionally the maxillary cuspids. Such teeth are designated *impacted teeth.*

Delay in shedding the deciduous teeth and eruption of the permanent teeth accompanied by the presence of supernumerary teeth and failure of the bones of the face, the skull, and the clavicle to develop properly is a hereditary mesodermal dysplasia, *cleidocranial dysostosis.* The presence of some deciduous teeth, a few permanent teeth, and absence of other teeth in an individual who has reached his late teens is very suggestive of this condition. Radiographs will demonstrate the presence of supernumerary teeth and the failure of the bones to develop.

Dilaceration is a condition in which the long axes of the crown and root are not in the same plane. The long axis of the root forms an angle with the long axis of the crown. This deviation of the root is usually due to crowding of the teeth during development, or it may be due to a blow which displaces the crown when root formation is beginning. The root continues to form in the original axis, while the crown remains in the displaced position.

"Dens in dente" is an anomalous development from invagination

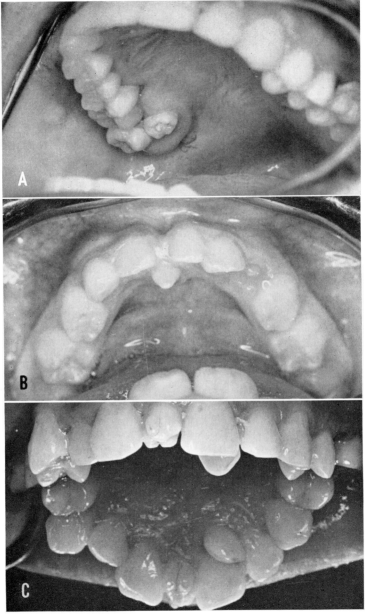

Figure 30. A, Supernumerary molar erupted palatal to third molar. B, Absence of one lateral incisor and presence of a mesiodens. C, Two supernumerary teeth: the one between the central incisors is called a mesiodens, and the one between the central and lateral incisors a distodens.

of the enamel into the area of a natural pit or groove. It most often occurs in the maxillary lateral incisors as an invagination of the enamel into the lingual pit. The enamel invagination may extend a short distance or to the apex of the root. Radiographically, the radiopaque enamel of the crown is continuous with enamel surrounding a central space. With enamel on both the outside and inside of the tooth, it has the appearance of a tooth within a tooth (Fig. 31). These teeth are frequently lost early owing to organisms or debris passing through the central space to the apical area where an inflammatory process is initiated similar to that which develops at the apex of a tooth with pulp disease.

Disturbances in the *position* of teeth may be caused by insufficient space on the arch for the size of the teeth which results in crowding, especially of anterior teeth. In some instances, there may be transposition of teeth (Fig. 32), i.e., the positions of the lateral incisor and cuspid may be reversed. Anomalous position of teeth may affect the esthetics of the teeth and the physiognomy of the individual to the extent that it is desirable to correct the position by orthodontic procedures.

Teeth may be too large (giantism) or too small (dwarfism). Giantism (Fig. 33) may involve all of the teeth, pairs of teeth, or the crown or root of a single tooth. Dwarfism involves the teeth

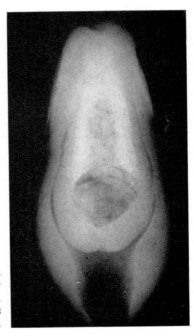

Figure 31. *"Dens in dente."* Incisor with enamel lining a central cavity extending to apex of root. A configuration of a tooth appears to be within the pulp chamber.

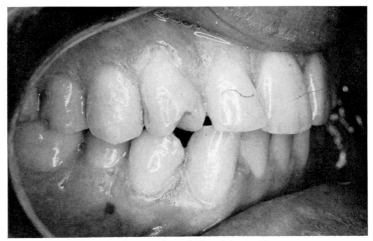

Figure 32. Transposition of cuspid and first bicuspid.

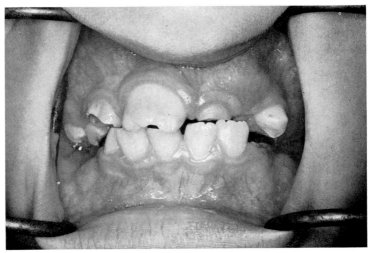

Figure 33. *Giantism.* Marked variation in size of teeth. The permanent central incisor is three times the width of the deciduous central incisor.

similarly but is more common than giantism. Most often third molars and maxillary lateral incisors are dwarfed. Dwarfed teeth frequently are abnormal in shape, especially the lateral incisor which may be represented as only a small peg-shaped tooth called a *"peg lateral"* (Fig. 34).

Disturbances in the *formation* of teeth occur at any stage of odontogenesis and involve any of the developing cellular components. Some defects in tooth development are genetic in origin and there-

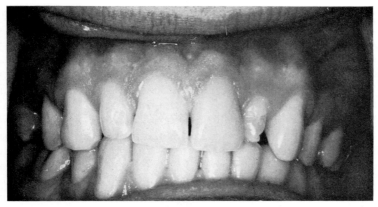

Figure 34. *"Peg Lateral."* Both maxillary lateral incisors are narrow; the left incisor is conical and shows hypoplasia of enamel.

fore usually involve all teeth and both dentitions. Such defects may be associated with dysplastic processes in other tissues developing from the same germ layer.

Amelogenesis imperfecta is a hereditary disturbance of enamel formation associated with other evidences of ectodermal dysplasia. This disturbance, which involves all teeth in both dentitions, is the result of a defect in the formation of the enamel matrix and the calcification and maturation of enamel. The severity of the defect in the formation of enamel varies in different patients, different teeth, and even different areas of the same tooth. Thus, the clinical appearance is rarely duplicated, although the basic defect of the enamel is the same in all cases. The characteristic findings are due to a failure of the formation of enamel matrix of one or more teeth or a portion of a tooth. The complete absence of enamel matrix results in teeth having the shape, size, and yellow color of the dentin core. Some variation in color is produced by staining from substances taken into the mouth. In teeth where areas of the enamel matrix is formed but not calcified, the surface of the defective enamel has a normal contour, but the enamel has a yellowish color and a soft, chalky consistency. In other areas the enamel is calcified and mature, so the enamel is normal in color and consistency. In spite of the poor formation of a portion of the enamel, such teeth have a low caries susceptibility and are not subject to marked attrition. However, these teeth are esthetic problems and, because of this, may cause psychologic problems necessitating the replacement or crowning of most of the teeth.

Another inherited disturbance of the enamel is *hereditary brown hypoplasia*. This defect involves the entire dentition uniformly and is due to a failure of maturation of normally formed enamel matrix. The teeth are normal in shape, size, and contour, but are altered in color and consistency. The teeth are the brownish-yellow color of immature enamel matrix and the consistency is about that of chalk. The patients are usually immune to caries, and attrition is slight even though the enamel is soft. These patients have a marked tendency for abundant calculus formation at early ages with the calculus being about the same color and consistency as the immature enamel. Removal of the calculus without disturbing the poorly calcified and poorly matured enamel is difficult. Because the teeth of patients with hereditary brown hypoplasia are uniform in appearance, they do not present esthetic problems as severe as does amelogenesis imperfecta. Esthetic and psychologic attitudes, however, do present problems which are solved in the same manner as in amelogenesis imperfecta.

Enamel hypoplasia is a disturbance in the formation of the enamel matrix from a variety of causes, resulting in defective enamel of one or several teeth. The hypoplastic defects vary in size, shape, and severity depending upon the etiology of the hypoplasia and the degree of tooth development reached at the time the defect was initiated. Hypoplasia is usually manifest as a series of irregular to round pits of varying size in the enamel (Fig. 35). The pits are frequently arranged in a row parallel to the incisal or coronal surfaces of the labial or lingual surfaces of the teeth. They follow the pattern of the imbrication lines. When the defect occurs in several teeth, it follows the chronologic pattern of tooth development. For example, hypoplastic defects may be present on the incisal one-third of the central incisors and the incisal tips of the cuspids, whereas the lateral incisors are not involved. This variation in involvement is due to the difference in time at which the various teeth develop, viz., the formation of the enamel of the central incisors and cuspids occurs before that of the lateral incisor teeth. The defects are usually stained brown to black. No particular immunity or susceptibility to caries is associated with enamel hypoplasia.

Hypoplasia may be caused by high fever, acute infectious diseases characterized by a rash (measles, chicken pox), dietary deficiencies, irradiation, local or generalized infection, or the ingestion of toxic substances. The nature of the defect is not always characteristic of a particular etiology; however, hypoplasia of the enamel can be correlated with a specific cause if the patient's history indicates that an etiologic factor was present during the time the defective parts of the teeth were being formed. In some cases, the type of defect is characteristic of a particular disease, such as syphilis or periapical infection of a deciduous tooth.

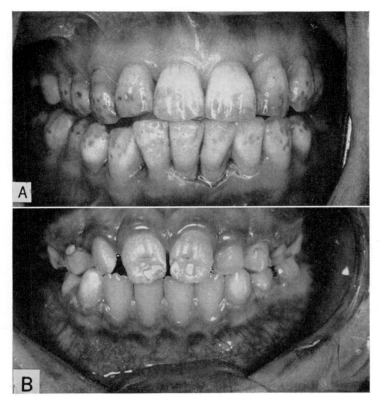

Figure 35. *Hypoplasia of enamel.* A, Nearly all teeth show hypomaturation of enamel and numerous small hypoplastic pits. B, Hypoplastic defects on incisal one-third of maxillary central incisors (no other teeth involved).

In congenital syphilis, hypoplasia may involve the maxillary central incisors and the first permanent molars. The incisors have a notch in the incisal edge and a mesio-distal narrowing of the incisal portion of the crown. This produces a shape like the notched blade of a screw driver (Fig. 36A, C). Such incisors are called *Hutchinson incisors* and are very suggestive but not positive evidence of congenital syphilis. Involved molars have a slight constriction of the occlusal surface which is composed of small nodular masses of enamel simulating the surface of a raspberry or mulberry and therefore are designated mulberry molars (also Pfluger molars) (Fig. 36B, C). Often the small nodular masses of enamel are poorly attached to the dentin and fracture away exposing the dentin of most of the occlusal surface. The appearance of the molars, like

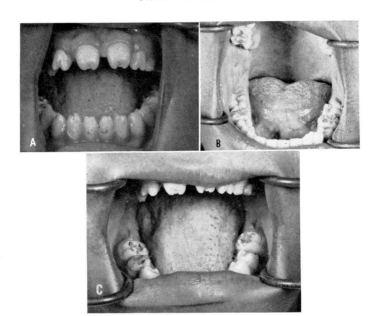

Figure 36. A, *Hutchinson's incisors*. Maxillary central incisors are typical and are usually the only teeth involved. However, the lower incisors are also affected in this instance. B, *Mulberry molars*. Both lower first molars show the small nodules of enamel resembling the surface of a berry. C, Hutchinson's incisors and mulberry molars.

that of the incisors, is very suggestive but not positive evidence of congenital syphilis.

When the pulp of a deciduous tooth is diseased, the presence of a periapical lesion may involve a part of the enamel organ of the succedaneous tooth and produce a defect in a limited area of the developing enamel of a permanent tooth. In this case, there is a defect involving a portion of a single surface of a single tooth (Fig. 37). Teeth so involved are characteristic and are named *Turner's teeth* after the investigator who first reported their occurrence and etiology.

Fluorosis or *mottled enamel* is a particular type of hypoplasia produced by the ingestion of water containing more than two parts per million of fluorine during the time when the enamel was forming. The fluorine incorporated into the forming enamel prevents its complete maturation and produces an opacity and porosity to the enamel (Fig. 38). The enamel is irregularly whitish-gray to brown with some exaggeration of the lines of imbrication. Mottled teeth are immune to caries, but are susceptible to enamel fracture and attrition. The loss of enamel with exposure of dentin sometimes

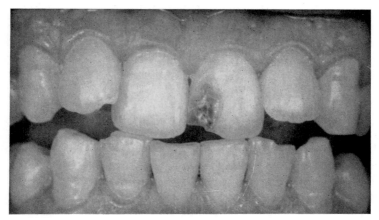

Figure 37. *Turner's tooth.* Focal hypoplasia of a portion of labial enamel of central incisor.

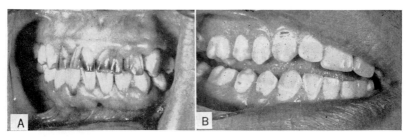

Figure 38. *Mottled enamel.* A, Some opacity and incisal wear with cracking and dark-brown staining of enamel. B, Patchy white mottling due to intense hypomaturation of enamel.

causes the teeth to become hypersensitive. Enamel fluorosis or mottling may be severe and unattractive but usually presents no esthetic problems in localities where it is common or endemic; however, mottled enamel does present a problem in individuals who move to a locality where it is uncommon. To overcome hypersensitivity and to improve the esthetic appearance, mottled teeth may have to be extracted and replaced or covered by crowns.

Pigmentation of a developing dentition may occur as the result of a mother's ingestion of the antibiotic tetracycline during her pregnancy. Such pigmentation may involve both the primary and permanent dentitions. This disturbance is a frequent complication in cystic fibrosis. Mild pigmentation shows as a yellow discoloration at the cervical margins of the teeth (Fig. 39A). In severe pigmentation the entire dentition may be stained brown to bluish-violet (Fig.

39B). Depending on the stage of dental development, staining may involve only a portion of the dentition.

Disturbances in dentin formation may accompany those produced in enamel, but are usually not clinically evident because they are hidden by the enamel covering the crowns. *Dentinogenesis imperfecta* is a mesodermal defect of hereditary character involving the dentin of the entire dentition (Fig. 40). Such dentin is poorly formed and contains less calcium salts, has a deeper color, and is more elastic in consistency than normal dentin. This alteration of the dentin gives the teeth an opalescent quality, there is a marked tendency for attrition, and the teeth may be worn away almost as fast as they erupt. The rate of dentinogenesis is so increased that the pulp chamber may be obliterated as the tooth forms. In radiographs, the teeth appear devoid of pulp chamber or root canals, and the roots appear blunted and narrow.

In *dentin dysplasia,* another defect of the dentin, the crowns of the

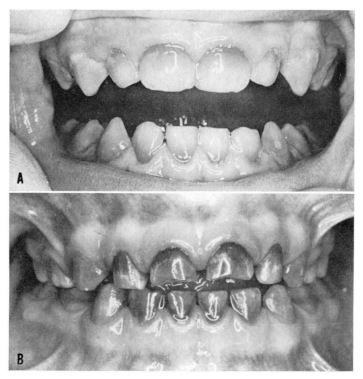

Figure 39. *Tetracycline pigmentation.* A, Mild effect with yellow to brownish pigmentation showing at the cervical one-third of the teeth. B, Intense effect with the entire tooth discolored. Note distribution is the same as A with greatest intensity at the cervical margins.

teeth appear normal in shape and color. The teeth are usually malposed owing to distorted, blunt, or absent roots. The pulp chambers are frequently absent, and there are rarefied areas in the bone at the apex of the peculiarly shaped roots. Radiographically, the rarefied areas resemble periapical cysts (Fig. 41).

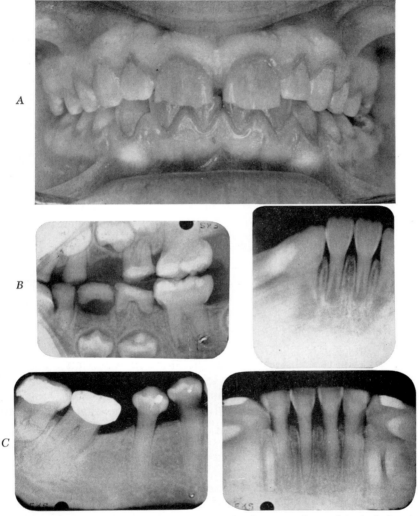

Figure 40. *Dentinogenesis imperfecta.* A, Opalescent color and incisal abrasion. B, Radiographs of erupted deciduous and developing permanent teeth showing obliteration of pulp chamber and extensive occlusal wear. C, Radiographs of permanent teeth of same patient ten years later showing characteristic configuration of root and obliteration of pulp chamber.

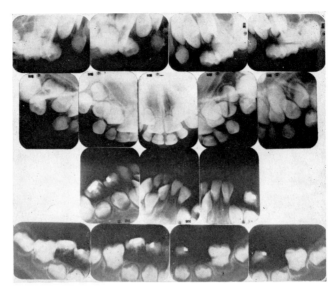

Figure 41. *Dentin dysplasia*—typical findings. Both dentitions are involved and show limited root formation with periapical radiolucency. The molar roots are square and show no tendency for bifurcation. The pulp chambers are absent.

Disturbances in cementum may occur, but are very rare and are not clinically discernible. When present, they are associated with premature shedding of the teeth.

Concrescence is the union of two teeth by cementum (Fig. 42). It most frequently occurs in the maxillary molar region between the second and third molars with the third molar in an abnormal position so that the roots of the teeth are in close contact. Excess deposition of cementum about malposed teeth fuses the roots together. They present a considerable problem in extraction because the condition is not evident clinically or by x-ray film examination.

Enamel pearls are small masses of enamel or dentin covered by enamel and are attached to the surface of the root. These malformations most often occur in the bifurcation of multi-rooted teeth as small (1 to 4 millimeters) globular masses of enamel partially covered by cementum (Fig. 43). They are formed by persistent amelogenic activity of a localized area of Hertwig's sheath. The enamel pearl may present a problem in the treatment of a periodontal pocket that has extended beyond the attachment of the enamel pearl.

During development, a single enamel organ may divide partially to form a tooth appearing to have two crowns (geminism). This

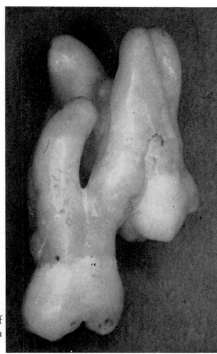

Figure 42. *Concrescence.* Fusion of roots by excess deposition of cementum.

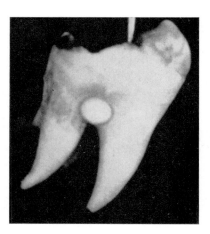

Figure 43. *Enamel pearl.*

defect may occur only as an incisal notch. Radiographs of geminism show that a single root and pulpal canal are present (Fig. 44). The normal number of teeth are present counting the divided crown as one. *Fusion* is a malformation produced by the union of two

6

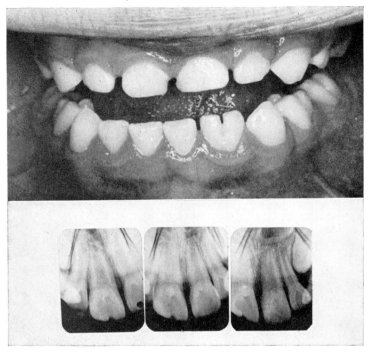

Figure 44. *Geminism. Upper,* Almost complete division of crown. Radiographs
show there is a common root. *Lower,* Radiographs of maxillary central incisors showing slight division of crown with common root.

developing adjacent teeth. Fusion occurs most often when a normal
tooth becomes fused with a supernumerary tooth. Radiographs of
fusion show a double root with two pulp canals.

BIBLIOGRAPHY

Colby, R. A., Kerr, D. A., and Robinson, H. B. G.: *Color Atlas of Oral Pathology,* 2nd ed. Philadelphia, J. B. Lippincott Co., 1961.

Lassi, A., and Partin, P.: The inheritance pattern of missing, peg-shaped and
strongly mesio-distally reduced upper lateral incisors. Acta Odont. Scand.,
27:563, 1969.

Lyons, C. J.: Etiology of cleft palate and cleft lip and some fundamental principles in operative procedure. J. Amer. Dent. Ass., 17:827, 1930.

Sanders, J.: Inheritance of harelip and cleft palate. Genetica, 15:433, 1934.

Shafer, G. G., Hine, M. K., and Levy, B. M.: *Textbook of Oral Pathology.*
Philadelphia, W. B. Saunders Co., 1958.

Stewart, D. J.: The effects of tetracyclines upon the dentition. Brit. J. Derm.,
76:374, 1964.

• Chapter 4

REACTION TO INJURY

INFLAMMATION

Inflammation is a nonspecific reaction of tissue to injury caused by mechanical, thermal, electrical, chemical, or bacterial agents. When tissue is crushed, torn, burned, or invaded by microorganisms, a protective reaction occurs in the tissue to limit the effects of the injury and to repair the damage. An inflammatory reaction to injury is a physiologic response of tissue which permits an organism to survive despite the almost constant destruction of many of its cells. This nonspecific response of the tissues should not be thought of as disease but should be considered as a favorable response of a part of the body to disease.

The presence of inflammation is designated by the suffix *-itis* attached to an anatomic designation of the part of the body injured. Thus, if there is inflammation of the appendix, it is appendicitis; if of the skin, dermatitis; and when the gingiva is involved, it is gingivitis. The latter is discussed in detail in Chapter 11, page 227.

The response of the body to injury is a very complex one and consists of an alteration of blood vessels, the mobilization of the cells of defense, the action of chemical (humoral) substances, and the formation of new tissue. These responses have been arbitrarily divided into the alterative, exudative, and reparative phases of inflammation, although no actual division of the process occurs.

The initial response of the tissue to an injury is a change in the diameter of the blood vessels of the injured area. Initially a constriction of the vessels occurs following injury which lasts for twenty to thirty seconds; then a gradual increase in size of the vessels occurs until they are larger than before injury. The increase in diameter of the vessels permits more blood to flow into the area of injury (active hyperemia) and decreases the rate of flow of blood through the vessels. As the rate of flow decreases, the white cells normally occupying the center of the stream of blood are forced toward the periphery of the stream where they appear to adhere to the walls of the vessels (margination).

In addition to dilatation of the vessels, there is an alteration in the permeability of the walls of the vessels allowing the fluids of the blood to pass into the the surrounding tissues and to accumulate in the intracellular spaces. The accumulation of fluid is called *edema.* When the white blood cells (leukocytes) make contact with the vessel walls, they emigrate through the walls into the intercellular spaces (Fig. 45). The movement of white cells through the walls of vessels is permitted by the altered permeability of the blood vessels and by the ability of the white cells to move by changing their shape (amoeboid movement). The white cells accumulate in the intercellular spaces along with the fluid that escaped from the vessels. The fluid and cells are designated an *exudate,* and the process by which they pass through the walls of the vessels into the tissue spaces is called *exudation.*

As the above alterations occur in the tissue following injury, recognizable changes are produced in the exposed parts. These changes, the cardinal signs of inflammation, include: (1) redness, (2) swelling, (3) heat, and (4) pain. These signs of inflammation vary in intensity with different types of injury. All are present to some degree in every response of the tissues to injury.

The redness associated with inflammation occurs because more blood (active hyperemia) is carried into the area of injury owing to

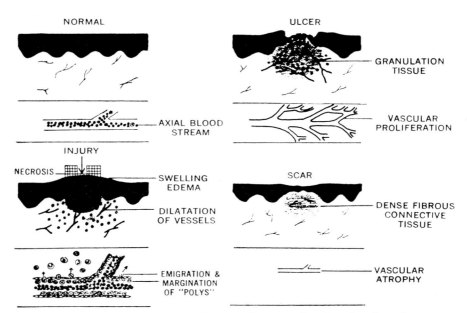

Figure 45. *Reaction to injury.* Schematic drawing showing the alterative, exudative, and reparative phases of inflammation.

the increase in size of the blood vessels. When near the surface, the red color of the blood shows through the skin or mucous membrane covering. Almost everyone is familiar with the redness of the skin that follows contact with a hot object, overexposure to sunlight, or the "inflamed" appearance of skin that occurs when microorganisms have invaded the tissue (infection).

The swelling that occurs following injury is produced as a result of the accumulation of fluid and cells which passed through the vessels into the intercellular spaces. This accumulation of fluid and cells pushes the tissue cells further apart and increases the bulk of the tissue. In some instances, when fluid accumulates near the surface of the skin or mucosa, the surface epithelium is elevated to produce a blister (vesicle). Blister formation is seen following burns from heat, sun, or friction.

The increase in temperature at the site of an injury is related to the presence of a greater than usual amount of blood in the area owing to the dilatation of vessels and an increase in the number of capillaries in use at one time in the area. The elevation of temperature can be recognized by placing the hand or a thermometer on the area of redness, viz., the feeling of heat related to areas of sunburn. All areas of redness due to hyperemia associated with injury are warmer than normal areas.

The pain of inflammation, not directly related to nerve injury and toxins, is associated with swelling. When the tissue spaces are filled with fluid and cells, excessive pressure is built up and is transmitted to nerve endings as a noxious and painful stimulus.

Simultaneously with the development of the clinical signs of inflammation, changes of a protective nature occur within the tissue. These changes are in part chemical and in part cellular. The accumulated fluid in the tissue spaces contains such chemical substances as *lysins*, which liquefy injured cells or bacteria; *antitoxins*, which neutralize toxins introduced into the tissue by the injurious agent or produced by organs introduced at the time of injury; *precipitins*, which precipitate substances into the tissues; and *agglutinins*, which have the ability to cause scattered microorganisms to be drawn into clumps. These and similar substances accumulated at the site of injury are all directed toward reducing the extent of injury. This form of defense, in which the substances are provided from the blood or the tissue fluid, is designated the humoral defense of the body. In addition, the escaped blood plasma contains fibrin, the element that makes the blood clot when it is outside of the blood vessels.

The *reticuloendothelial system* is a widespread cellular system consisting of reticulum cells in the spleen and lymph nodes, and endothelial cells lining capillaries of the liver, spleen, and lymph nodes. Also included in this system are wandering reticuloendothelial cells, histiocytes and monocytes, which are macrophages. Polymorphonuclear leukocytes, lymphocytes, and plasma cells are also considered to be part of the R-E system. The functions of this system are related to cellular and humoral defense of the body: phagocytosis and the formation of antibodies.

The reaction of the R-E system to substances of a protein nature and cellular species usually occurs in a specific way. The system responds to the introduction of a protein that is foreign to the body by the formation of substances capable of destroying or inactivating the disease-producing agent. The foreign agent is termed an *antigen,* and the substances formed in response to this agent are called *antibodies* or immune bodies. Nonprotein substances may combine with proteins to form antigens called partial antigens or *haptens.* The formation of antibodies generally is the result of an exposure to antigens. As a result of the exposure and the development of immune bodies, a complete or partial immunity to the antigens is present. In this way a specialized state of resistance is developed, viz., immunity to contracting measles or smallpox after having had the disease.

Immunity may be natural or acquired. Natural immunity is essentially genetic in origin and is relatively permanent. Thus immunologic responses, the reaction of antibodies to potential pathologic agents, occur in an individual who has not had the disease related to the pathogens nor received artificially produced immunity (immunization). Natural immunity may be species specific; humans are immune to certain diseases that occur in animals. Acquired immunity may occur naturally as the result of having had a disease in either mild or severe form. This type of acquired immunity is considered to be actively acquired immunity. An immunity may be acquired artificially in a passive or active way. Artificial passive immunity is acquired by the injection of antiserum, whereas active immunity is acquired by vaccination with live, dead, or attenuated organisms. A smallpox vaccination results in an active immunity, but such immunity does not last as long as that acquired naturally (following the disease). Active immunity lasts longer than passive immunity, but takes much longer to develop. An artificially acquired passive immunity occurs very rapidly following the injection of an immunizing serum (sterile serum obtained from an individual or animal carrying antibodies naturally or artificially produced). An immunizing serum is usually given as a therapeutic or prophylactic measure when an individual already has a sickness or when the danger of contracting a disease is imminent during an epidemic.

Disturbances in the immune response may result in *autoimmune* and autoimmune-like diseases. Examples of such disturbances include anaphylaxis, allergy, erythroblastosis fetalis (Rh factor incompatibility), rheumatoid arthritis, and ulcerative colitis. These diseases occur in part or whole because of antigen-antibody reactions. It is not clear why the organism has or develops antibodies which are destructive to itself in autoimmune diseases. The production of antibodies in response to an organism's own tissues (tissue antigens) with resulting tissue damage is one of the foremost challenges in immunology. Also of special interest at this time is the artificial repression of immune responses for the purpose of organ transplants and the rejection of transplants at some time after the transplant operation.

There is some experimental evidence to suggest a relationship between periodontal disease and local immunologic injury to the periodontium. The presence of serum antibodies directed against oral bacteria, localization of immunoglobulins in inflamed gingiva, and the presence of numerous plasma cells (which arise in response to antigenic stimulation) in periodontal inflammation suggest the possibility that hypersensitivity reactions may play a role in the tissue injury associated with periodontal disease.

The same mechanism that produces blood clotting causes the coagulation of edema fluid by precipitation of fibrin to consolidate the area and block lymphatic drainage. The solidification of the fibrin and the blocking of lymphatic drainage prevent diffusion of microorganisms and chemical substances from the area of injury. The precipitation of fibrin causes the area of swelling to become firm rather than soft as when it is filled with fluid.

As the vessel undergoes dilatation and the blood flow decreases, the white cells marginate and contact the endothelial lining of the vessel. The same alteration in a vessel wall which permits the escape of fluid now permits the white blood cells to pass through the wall (emigration) into the tissue spaces. The first cell to negotiate the wall is the polymorphonuclear cell which, because of its ability to carry out amoeboid movement, is capable of passing through the now permeable wall and of migrating along fibrin strands to the area of tissue injury. A substance (leukotoxine) is liberated, providing a chemical attraction for the leukocytes. The chemical attraction of the leukocytes to the area of alteration is called chemotaxis and provides for a concentration of leukocytes in the area of injury to participate in the resolution of the injury. In addition to the local influence at the site of injury, a systemic response is apparent in significant inflammatory reactions and is indicated by an increase in the number of leukocytes in the peripheral blood.

The first cell to reach the area of injury is the polymorphonuclear neutrophilic leukocyte or neutrophil (Fig. 46). The neutrophil is produced by the bone marrow and circulates in the blood for about

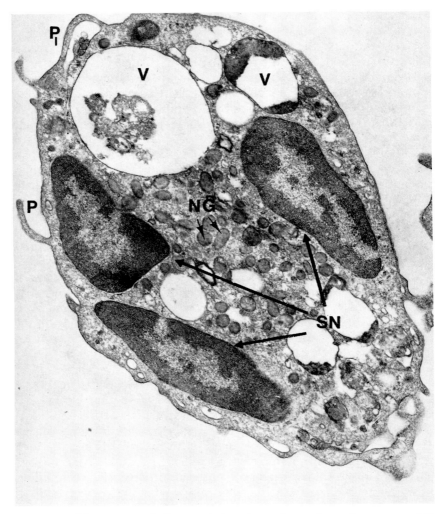

Figure 46. *Ultrastructural characteristics of a polymorphonuclear neutrophilic leukocyte.* The segmented nuclei (SN) are present, but the linking nucleoplasm is not present in this section. Numerous neutrophilic granules (NG) are present throughout the cytoplasm. Large vacuoles (V) are seen which may represent the residual elements of phagocytized material. The peripheral cytoplasm is specialized into projections (P) which fold over and re-unite with the cytoplasm to capture material (P$_1$). Magnification approximately × 10,000. (Courtesy of Dr. David Krutchoff.)

21 days after which it dies and is replaced by a new cell. By this process a constant supply of highly viable cells is available for defense of the body. The neutrophils carry out important functions at the site of injury. These cells are capable of ingesting and digesting certain microorganisms by a process known as *phagocytosis.* The destruction of microorganisms by phagocytosis is one of the most important protective functions of the body against the spread of microorganisms and the initiation of infection. Because these cells are the first to reach the area of injury and because of their ability to destroy microorganisms, they are designated the "first line of defense."

Upon death the neutrophil liberates a proteolytic enzyme responsible for the digestion of microorganisms and liquefaction of the injured tissue and fibrin which was precipitated in the area of injury. By destroying microorganisms, preventing infection, and liquefying the fibrin and debris, the cells play an important role in the resolution of the area of injury.

Other white blood cells having a function in the inflammatory response are the *monocytes* (macrophages). These cells are transported from bone marrow to the site of injury. Other cells of identical appearance and function develop at the site of alteration (fixed phagocytes). The cells are capable of phagocytosis and engulf microorganisms other than cocci, particulate matter of small and large size introduced at the time of injury, and the debris of cells killed at the time of injury. Because of their small size and their ability to ingest only small microorganisms, the neutrophils are designated *microphages;* the larger mononuclear cells, which can digest larger microorganisms and particulate matter, are designated *macrophages.*

When in contact with particles larger than themselves, the macrophages fuse together to produce large multinucleated cells called *foreign body giant cells.* The foreign body is surrounded by the combined cytoplasm of several cells permitting destruction of the mass by the enlarged cell. These cells, because of their late arrival at the site of injury and the nature of their function, are designated the "second line of defense."

Another type of white blood cell participating in the inflammatory reaction is the *lymphocyte,* a product of lymphoid tissue that is transported by the blood to the area of injury. These cells are composed almost entirely of nuclear material and provide a rich source of nuclear proteins for the rebuilding of the injured tissue. These cells serve to produce antibodies, and when functioning in this capacity, change their histologic features and are designated plasma cells. They produce large molecular proteins in the range of globulins which appear to be the antibodies. By formation of antibodies, these cells participate in the humoral defense of the body.

Some of the polymorphonuclear cells contain granules with an affinity for certain dyes. Those having an affinity for acidophilic dyes are called eosinophils, and those having an affinity for basic dyes are designated as basophils.

The *eosinophils* appear in allergic reactions and injuries owing to foreign proteins and parasites. The cells produce histamine or some similar anti-inflammatory substance. The *basophil* is found in inflammatory responses characterized by the presence of abundant edema fluid. Since consolidation would inhibit the resolution of the injurious reaction, the basophils inhibit consolidation of the area of alteration by producing anticoagulant heparin or some closely related substance. The combined action of the various white cells makes up the first and second lines of defense and is the cellular defense which complements the humoral defense in overcoming the effects of injury.

The combined action of the humoral and cellular defenses through continued liquefaction of tissue debris, the phagocytosis of microorganisms and foreign material, and the neutralization of various substances by antibodies prepare the way for the third phase of the inflammatory reaction—repair.

Once the humoral and cellular defenses have limited the effects of the injurious agent to the immediate area of injury, the cellular defenses are directed toward the removal of dead bacteria, white cells, and necrotic tissue. Upon the death of the neutrophils (microphages) at the site of injury, enzymes are liberated into the tissues that digest the fibrin precipitated from the tissue fluid as well as dead cells and bacteria in the area. At the same time macrophages are ingesting cellular debris and foreign material. The liquefaction of the fibrin, dead cells, and bacteria, and the elimination of the cell debris by the macrophages cause the area of injury to soften and become fluid in character. This liquefied material, which contains large numbers of dead neutrophils and cell debris, is *pus*. The process of forming pus is called *suppuration*. An *abscess* is the accumulation of pus in a localized area. If an abscess develops near the surface of the skin or mucosa, the accumulated pus may escape or drain to the exterior and thereby provide for rapid elimination of the dead material. If the pus is deep in the tissues and cannot escape, the fluid portion diffuses into the blood vessels and lymphatics to be carried from the site of injury to other parts of the body for complete destruction. An extensive accumulation of pus in the facial spaces associated with pulp disease and an alveolar abscess may require surgical incision and drainage. With continuous liquefaction and phagocytosis all of the debris ultimately is eliminated from the area and the injured cells can be replaced by new ones (healing). If the tissue injury is minimal, the dead cells are destroyed and replaced without pus formation. However, certain organisms characteristically produce suppuration and are called pyogenic (pus-producing) bacteria.

Inflammation may be of different types depending upon the tissue affected and the nature of the injury. Each tissue has a different reactive capacity dictated by the structure and function of the tissue or organ. Each etiologic factor also elicits a specific or typical response in the tissue injured. It is therefore significant to be aware of the types of reactions which occur in various tissues in response to particular types of injury. Having this information one can recognize the nature of an inflammatory response and know that a specific etiologic factor is producing the typical reaction. The specific reaction of a tissue to a specific injury is designated a disease entity. For example, a swelling of the parotid gland produced by a specific virus is designated mumps. Because there are so many typical reactions to specific factors which are given names indicating a disease entity, we are apt to think that the inflammatory response is pathologic rather than physiologic.

Basic types of inflammatory response are indicated by the nature of the exudate produced and are designated accordingly. A *serous exudate* is due to an outpouring of a large amount of fluid in the early stage of the response. It is high in protein but low in fibrinogen. This process typically occurs in body cavities lined by serosa. It is the type of response produced by the pleura, the pericardium, and the peritoneum. In other responses there is abundant fluid but the fluid is high in fibrinogen so that fibrin is precipitated onto a tissue surface. Such an exudate is designated a *fibrinous exudate* and is seen in the same locations as serous exudates. If an exudate contains many red cells, it is a *sanguineous* or *hemorrhagic exudate*. This is produced when the permeability of the vessels is intense. *Mucinous* or *catarrhal exudates* are produced by tissues having the ability to produce mucin. Large quantities are produced by the cells to protect a body surface against irritants. It is seen in the respiratory and digestive tracts where the mucosa normally produces mucin and the physiologic capacity is exaggerated in response to mucosal injury. Upper respiratory infection with bronchitis is an excellent example of a catarrhal inflammation.

In injuries where the chemotactic effect is intense, numerous leukocytes are attracted to the area of alteration and produce a purulent inflammation. In situations where many of the polymorphonuclear cells die and liberate an enzyme capable of liquefying tissue, the process is called *suppuration* and the exudate pus. Boils, carbuncles, and abscesses are suppurative processes and are characterized by the presence of pus. Since cocci in an area of injury lead to the production of pus, such organisms are designated pus producing; the polymorphonuclear cells in this situation are designated as pus cells.

Purulent inflammation in some cases results in an intense liquefaction process and diffuse spread of the inflammation through the tissue and is called cellulitis or phlegmon. When mucosal surfaces are injured by highly toxic agents, intracellular coagulation necrosis results and abundant fibrin is precipitated in the necrotic tissue and on the surface to form a membrane-like covering to the area of injury. This process may be initiated by the toxin of the diphtheria bacilli. The process is diphtheritis and the covering membrane is a pseudo- or diphtheritis membrane. Such a pseudomembrane typifies diphtheria and ulceromembranous gingivitis (p. 228).

Any of the inflammatory responses may be present at various stages of activity. If only the alterative and exudative processes are present, the stage of inflammation is acute, the course is rapid, and the classical signs that are evident are often associated with sudden, intense constitutional symptoms. The process may subside or may progress to a subacute or chronic inflammation.

Subacute inflammation demonstrates active acute inflammation with some evidence of fibrous proliferation heralding the beginning of repair. It is an intermediate stage between acute and chronic.

Chronic inflammation is characterized by changes in which the alterative and exudative processes have been prolonged and proliferation of connective tissue is a prominent feature. The connective tissue formed shows evidence of maturity and the cellular response changes from the early accumulation of polymorphonuclear cells to one of an accumulation of later-arriving macrophages, lymphocytes, and plasma cells. The active proliferation of tissue is called productive inflammation.

HEALING: REPAIR AND REGENERATION

The passage through the various stages of inflammation is directed toward elimination of the altered tissue and exudate and the replacement of the injured cells either by connective tissue or by the same tissue as that destroyed. When tissue is replaced by connective tissue, the process is repair; when replaced by functional tissue of the type destroyed, it is regeneration. The resolution of the inflammatory response is healing—the goal of inflammation.

Repair

Fibroblastic and angioblastic proliferations are the fundamental tissue reaction in the repair of injury and result in replacement of injured cells. It is a specific cellular response following or occurring concomitantly with the vascular and exudative phase of the inflammatory reaction. The repair of tissue begins with a proliferation of

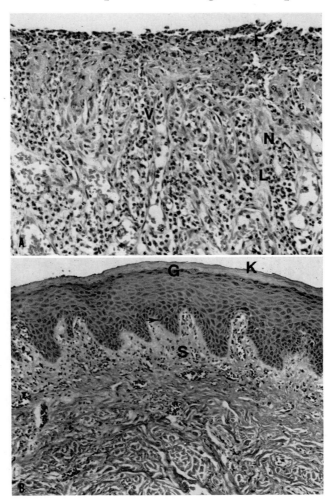

Figure 47. A, *Granulation tissue of an ulcer;* fibrin membrane with entrapped cell debris (F); newly formed vascular channels growing into fibrin (V); new fibroblasts (N); leukocytes (L), chiefly polymorphonuclear cells. B, *Mature scar* surfaced by hyperplastic hyperkeratotic epithelium; keratin layer (K), granular layer (G), division figure (→), maturing scar (S) in subepithelial layer.

angioblasts in thrombosed vessels at the border of the area of injury. Angioblasts proliferate through the thrombi and into the precipitated fibrin at the border of the exudate. As the proliferating angioblasts produce capillary buds, they are surrounded by proliferating fibroblasts. The invasion of blood clots or coagulated exudate by young vascular connective tissue is designated *organization,* and the highly vascular connective tissue (with associated inflammatory cells) is designated *granulation tissue* (Fig. 47A). The initial tissue of repair is then a delicate, highly vascular connective tissue. When a large quantity of granulation tissue is present, the reaction is termed a granulomatous response. In large defects, such as tuberculous cavities or large abscesses, the entire defect may not be filled with granulation tissue but only lined with granulation tissue. In such instances it is necessary to collapse the walls of the defect so that the walls can approximate and healing can occur.

When areas of skin are damaged, the base of the wound is filled with granulation tissue over which new squamous epithelium proliferates. Without a highly vascular bed of granulation tissue, epithelization will not occur. In very large wounds, skin grafts may be necessary to achieve complete healing.

When organization of the wound is complete and the defect has been filled with granulation tissue, the inflammatory cells slowly disappear and the capillaries decrease in size and number owing to replacement by fibrous tissue. The collagen fibers of the connective tissue become larger and more compact, which is evidence of maturity of the granulation tissue. Total maturation of granulation tissue results in a *scar* (Fig. 47B). Initially, the scar is a delicate, highly vascular connective tissue more than filling the defect. It gradually matures and contracts resulting in a dense, slightly vascular, pale area which may not completely replace the area of injury. An excess of granulation tissue may be present in some situations and is popularly referred to as "proud flesh." Excessive and continued production of scar results in a *keloid.* Where exudate fills body spaces and the area between two structures undergoes organization, union of the structure occurs and is called *adhesions.* Adhesions occur chiefly in the pericardial and pleural spaces, and the fixation by adhesions of the heart and lungs to the surrounding tissue produces both cardiac and pulmonary problems.

When the healing of a small, clean, uninfected wound (where the borders of the wound can be approximated) occurs with a minimum of granulation tissue, it is said to heal by *primary intention.* A larger wound without approximation of the borders will first be repaired by granulation tissue and then replaced by scar or covered by regenerated epithelium. When healing is preceded by the formation of granulation tissue, it is said to be by *secondary intention*. The granulation tissue must be built up slowly from the bottom and sides of the wound so that the epithelium will have a good vascular bed over which to regenerate.

The effectiveness of the healing process is determined by a variety of factors. Optimal healing is accomplished when an adequate supply of protein in the diet is accompanied by vitamins C and D. Calcium salts in the proper proportion to vitamin D are necessary for bone repair. Some factors delaying healing include: mechanical, chemical, or bacterial injury; foreign bodies, such as suture material, metals, silicon, cotton fiber, and calculus; and ACTH or cortisone.

The changes that take place in healing can be easily observed in injuries near the surface of the body. As resolution of the injury occurs and the injured area is replaced by granulation tissue, the redness and swelling are reduced and the tissue is of nearly normal consistency and color; however, the area of injury is still discernible. Gradually, however, the zone of injury becomes smaller, the tissue less red and more firm. Ultimately it becomes paler and firmer than the surrounding tissue because of a reduction of vascular channels and the denseness of the mature connective tissue. This mature area of repair is called a scar (Fig. 47B). A scar is the landmark of previous injury and its repair. The abundance of scar is proportionate to the degree of injury. Resolution of all injury is accomplished by repair, which is the replacement of the damaged cells by connective tissue.

Regeneration

In contrast to repair is the process of regeneration which means the replacement of areas of injury by the same type of tissue present in the area previous to the injury. Each type of cell possesses different ability to undergo reproduction. Some cells reproduce rapidly to almost unlimited degree, whereas others reproduce slowly or not at all. The cells of blood vessels and connective tissue form most rapidly and thus initially repair an area of injury; this tissue may be replaced later by more slowly growing and more highly specialized tissue. Surface epithelium forms almost as rapidly as connective tissue and blood vessels so that as the base of a surface wound heals, new epithelium begins to grow over the surface (Fig. 48). If cells of more highly specialized tissues, such as nerves, glands, and muscles, are present at the border of a zone of injury, they will grow into the area of repair to form new nerves, glands, or muscle tissues; this is *regeneration*. If all of the more specialized cells are destroyed, regeneration does not occur and the area of injury is replaced only by scar tissue.

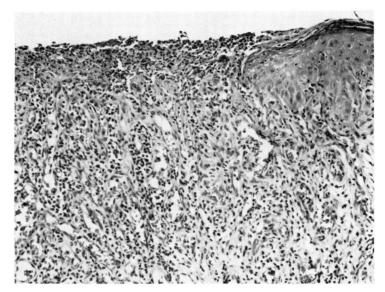

Figure 48. *Granulation tissue* at the border of a healing ulcer. *Regenerating epithelium* at upper right.

The capacity for regeneration is dependent on the size of the area injured, the presence or absence of infection, the age and nutritional state of the individual, and the degree of specialization of the tissue. The more highly specialized the tissue, the less possibility of regeneration. Connective tissue, blood vessels, surface epithelium, and blood-forming tissue have a marked ability to regenerate. Nerves, bone, and cartilage have moderate ability, but glands, smooth, voluntary, and cardiac muscle, as well as the central nervous system have almost no ability to regenerate. The same factors which influence healing also govern regeneration.

Our discussion indicates that inflammation is an altruistic nonspecific response of the body directed toward localizing injury so that injurious agents do not extend to wider and wider areas and ultimately destroy the entire body. Without such a reaction, the individual could not survive for long in an environment in which injury is so constant an occurrence. On some occasions the injury is so extreme or overwhelming that the response is inadequate and the death of the individual occurs.

INFECTION

Infection is the reaction of the tissue to invasion and injury by microorganisms. The mere presence of microorganisms on the surface of tissues does not mean infection; infection is present only when there is injury and a reaction of the body to the presence of implanted microorganisms.

The possibility of an infection developing is dependent upon the virulence, number, and type of organism; the capability of the organism for invading and surviving in the type of tissue involved; and the defense mechanism of the host. In addition to the defense mechanisms of the body described previously with inflammation, other natural body mechanisms of defense are present to inhibit the development of an infectious disease. These natural mechanisms of defense include certain enzymes of the saliva and tears, such as lysozyme, which are capable of inhibiting the growth of bacteria; the gastric juices, which are capable of destroying most organisms that are swallowed; the intact skin and mucosa with their secretions, which present an important barrier to bacterial growth and invasion; and natural antibodies, which contain antibacterial factors.

The effectiveness of these defense mechanisms vary considerably. Some of the factors predisposing an organism to infection are malnutrition, injury to the skin or mucosa, childhood or old age, and systemic diseases, such as diabetes mellitus.

Organisms not only enter the tissue, but when infected tissue is manipulated, the organisms may enter the blood stream without producing symptoms or tissue damage. Such a state is *bacteremia*. When the presence of organisms in the blood stream is accompanied by symptoms, such as chills and fever, the process is *septicemia*. When pyogenic organisms are spread by the blood to produce abscesses in many areas, the process is *pyemia*. Toxins produced by microorganisms may be transported by the blood to produce injury to specific tissues and is termed *toxemia*. A specific type of reaction to the products of particular organisms produces specific diseases of which diphtheria and tetanus are excellent examples. The discontinuous spread of microorganisms or the transportation of bacterial toxins to produce disease in an area remote from the initial site of infection is a *focal infection*. In diphtheria, where the organisms are in the pharynx, the toxins of these organisms produce cardiac damage and thus this disease is an excellent example of focal infection.

The body responds differently to each type of microorganism, and in many conditions the response is so characteristic that the reaction is indicated as a specific disease. There are many types of microorganisms to which there is a specific tissue reaction, whereas some organisms of the same type produce a nonspecific response. These organisms can be divided into the following groups: viruses, cocci, bacilli, spirochetes, and fungi.

7

Viruses

Viruses in general are much smaller than bacteria and are capable of survival only within living cells. Their needs for survival are very specific and as intracellular inhabitants they compete for the metabolites needed by the host cells. Thus, viruses have an affinity for certain types of tissue, such as nerve or skin, and always localize in a specific tissue regardless of how they enter the body. This affinity for specific tissue is called tropism, and the virus is said to be neurotropic when it localizes in nerve tissue or dermatotropic when it localizes in skin. Rabies and poliomyelitis are examples of diseases caused by neurotropic viruses. The viruses producing chicken pox, smallpox, or warts are dermatotropic viruses. The common cold and associated upper respiratory infections are viral in origin. The herpes simplex virus is a dermatotropic virus which produces the oral disease known as herpetic stomatitis discussed under stomatitis in Chapter 12, page 254. With the exception of the common cold and herpes, most specific viral infections are followed by long-lasting immunity.

Some of the more important viral diseases affect the central nervous system for which certain viruses (neurotropic) appear to have a marked affinity. One of the best known of the central nervous system viral diseases is poliomyelitis (infantile paralysis), an acute infection involving primarily the spinal cord and resulting in paralysis of muscles. The damage to the spinal cord is permanent, and since muscle function is never reestablished, muscle atrophy results. The recently developed "polio" vaccine is an effective preventive measure, and the incidence of the disease has been greatly reduced by its widespread use.

Rabies is a viral disease transmitted by the bite of a rabid (infected) animal, usually a dog. The virus is introduced into a bite wound by saliva containing the virus. The virus is neurotropic and localizes in brain tissue producing a disease (hydrophobia) that is always fatal unless early treatment is initiated. The disease is characterized by muscular spasm, excitement, convulsions, coma, and death.

Some viruses affect the respiratory tract and produce a variety of reactions recognized as the common cold, influenza, and pneumonia. Influenza is the most common of the pulmonary viral diseases. It is periodically epidemic and results in severe disease and death. In the 1918 epidemic millions of deaths resulted from the almost universal infection which occurred. The disease is an acute inflammation of the nasopharynx, trachea, and bronchioles. If the individual does not succumb to the initial infection, secondary infection by cocci and bacteria may result in pneumonia and cause death.

The skin also is a common site for viral localization and common acute infectious diseases result. *Smallpox* (variola) is an acute infectious process spread by droplets from the respiratory tract or by direct contact with an infected individual. The symptoms are high fever, severe headache, and vesicles which become invaded by streptococci to produce pustules. The disease remits spontaneously in two to three weeks or is fatal owing to streptococcal septicemia and secondary pneumonia. Having contracted the disease provides a lasting immunity. Smallpox can be prevented by vaccination.

Cocci

Cocci are small, round organisms which grow in irregular grapelike clusters or in chains and are gram-positive when stained with gram stain. There are two main types of pathogenic cocci: the staphylococci and the streptococci.

Staphylococci are natural inhabitants of the skin which are introduced into wounds or other areas of injury where they multiply and produce a strong exotoxin having an intense local necrotizing effect. Wherever the organisms gain a foothold and produce local necrosis, polymorphonuclear cells are attracted in large numbers to phagocytize the invaders. These cells in the area of liquefaction constitute pus, and the focal accumulation is an abscess. Because of this ability of the staphylococci to initiate pus production and abscess formation, they are termed pus-producing organisms. The invasion of a hair follicle or sebaceous gland duct by streptococci results in small abscesses called *furuncles* (pimples). They are very common on the face, especially with the development of the beard associated with the beginning of sexual maturity. Severe involvement of the entire face at this time is designated acne. More extensive infections associated with hair follicles where pus extends into the deeper subepithelial areas with a large area of necrosis is a *boil.* When the lesion involves many hair follicles and there are numerous areas of discrete necrosis and pus formation involving a large area, the lesion is a *carbuncle.* Staphylococci septicemia results from the hematogenous spread of these organisms from a localized focus to other areas producing multiple pyogenic abscesses. This condition may result in staphylococci nephritis, endocarditis, pneumonia, or osteomyelitis.

Streptococci are spherical organisms which grow in chains, possess a gram-positive staining reaction, and are hemolytic or anhemolytic, depending on the ability of the exotoxins to produce hemolysis. The reaction of the tissues to the streptococci is basically the same in all areas and the disease process is named according to anatomic site, viz., tonsillitis, pharyngitis, endocarditis, cellulitis, nephritis. Streptococci frequently localize in the pharynx and tonsillar area to produce "strep sore throat." The hemolytic streptococcus is the cause of bronchopneumonia, ulcerative endocarditis, scarlet fever, and erysipelas. The anhemolytic streptococci (Streptococcus viridans) produce subacute bacterial endocarditis when septicemia transports these organisms to previously injured heart valves. The avenue of invasion is often through the oral cavity following vigorous scaling or extraction of infected teeth. There is some question as to the part played by the streptococci in the production of rheumatic fever.

Other varieties of cocci are responsible for specific disease processes, such as lobar pneumonia due to pneumococci, meningitis due to meningococci, and gonorrhea due to gonococci.

It is apparent that this group of organisms (cocci) is responsible for a wide range of disease processes. It is this category of infection that is most effectively treated by antibiotics.

Bacilli

Bacilli are rod-shaped organisms of many varieties which produce widely different tissue reactions in many areas of the body. Bacilli are responsible for such disease processes as diphtheria, whooping cough, dysentery, tetanus, undulant fever, tularemia, tuberculosis, gingivitis, and dental caries. Dental caries are discussed in more detail in Chapter 9 and gingivitis in Chapter 11.

Diphtheria, whooping cough, and dysentery are acute infectious types of disease spread by droplets or by direct contact with infected individuals. They have specific symptom patterns and run short courses to terminate in spontaneous remission or death. Diphtheria and whooping cough are controlled well by immunization. Tetanus and gas gangrene are bacterial diseases in which the organisms gain entrance through wounds. The organisms are anaerobic and generally produce exotoxins responsible for characteristic tissue reactions.

Anthrax, plague, undulant fever, and tularemia are acute infectious processes in which the source of infection is wild or domestic animals. Each disease is produced by a specific type of bacillus and results in a distinct and characteristic response.

Tuberculosis is produced by a specific bacillus (tubercle bacillus) which, because of staining properties, is acid fast. Tuberculosis is widespread throughout the world, especially where there are concentrations of population living under urban conditions. Under these conditions it is often a progressive chronic disease which ultimately has a fatal termination. When introduced into isolated population groups, the individuals lack native resistance and the disease acts as an acute infectious disease with rapid fatal termination. This infection is spread by direct contact with persons having the disease. The disease also contaminates cattle, and milk obtained from infected animals produces the disease in man. Birds also are infected and avian tuberculosis may be transmitted to man.

The lung is the organ most often infected but the lymph nodes, intestine, kidney, brain, and bone, especially the spine, also are sites of infection. Pulmonary tuberculosis usually is acquired in childhood or early adult life owing to direct inhalation to the lungs of infected sputum or dust. Small infections may be overcome by the body defenses but initiate a sensitivity to the organisms so that subsequent infections produce severe disease. The body defenses are somewhat effective against the organisms so that the disease is slowly progressive with caseation necrosis produced by the exotoxins of the tuberculosis bacillus. The expanding necrosis initiates an intense inflammation with abundant characteristic granulation tissue surrounding areas of cavitation. The cavities are produced when the necrotic tissue is expelled through the bronchial tract by coughing. Spread from the lungs to other areas through the blood stream initiates infection in the brain, spine, joints, and some viscera.

Isolation of infected persons, prolonged rest treatment, and recently, chemotherapeutic agents have greatly reduced the prevalence of this disease. Tuberculosis of lymph nodes, stomach, and joints has been greatly reduced by the pasteurization of milk and the control of dairy herds.

Spirochetes

Spirochetes are small spiral forms of microorganisms which are somewhat motile. They produce a variety of diseases, the best known of which is *syphilis.* Syphilis has been a widespread venereal disease of great importance in medicine and dentistry, but with the development of penicillin the disease has been more effectively controlled and, to a certain degree, is no longer of great social or biologic importance so it will not be discussed in detail. Spirochetes also produce yaws, relapsing fever, rat bite fever, and fusospirochetal disease. Fusospirochetal disease results from the symbiotic relationship of a spirochete, Borrelia vincentii, and a fusiform bacillus. The gingival tissues are most frequently involved and the disease is called Vincent's infection or necrotizing ulcerative gingivitis, discussed in more detail under gingival disease in Chapter 11. Aspiration of the organisms during prolonged general anesthesia results in aspiration pneumonia.

Fungi

Fungi or mycotic organisms are cellular saprophytic or parasitic filamentous plants thus obtaining their food from dead organic material or living organisms. A variety of fungi produce a wide range of diseases in various parts of the body.

Because of their resistance to therapy, the mycoses are extremely chronic diseases. Infection of the skin is manifest as athlete's foot or candidiasis. Infection of the mucous membranes by the Candida albicans, a yeast-like organism, is thrush (p. 258). The fungi of the oral cavity most often responsible for oral diseases are candida and actinomyces. Candida albicans causes thrush and actinomyces (ray fungus) causes actinomycosis (lumpy jaw). Candida albicans is a yeast-like organism frequently present in the mouth without producing disease; however, when the resistance of the tissue is lowered, this fungus may enter the tissue and produce injury. Candida may also act to produce disease when a person has had extensive penicillin therapy which eliminates all other organisms and permits the unaffected candida to increase in number to the point of producing disease. Because of the widespread use of penicillin and similar antibiotics, candidiasis (thrush) is increasing in frequency.

In addition to the local reaction of the tissues to injury by infectious agents, clinical systemic signs and symptoms are generally evident. Such manifestations arise following a period of incubation, the period of time between local invasion of the tissues by microorganisms and the clinical manifestations of the infectious process. Following this period, which may be from hours to years, many infectious diseases exhibit prodromal symptoms of headache, malaise, and other minor disturbances. The onset of the full manifestations of the disease may occur abruptly or insiduously after the prodromal symptoms. It is during the full development of the infectious process that general manifestations occur such as fever, leukocytosis, chills, dehydration, increased heart rate, nervous symptoms, and decreased urinary output. Many of the infectious diseases have a rather characteristic onset, course, and subsidence; they are designated acute infectious diseases. Acute infectious diseases terminate rather abruptly with a complete cure, although in some cases complications may occur. Such diseases usually provide a lasting or permanent immunity. Other diseases do not mobilize such an intense and effective defense and thus are of a prolonged progressive nature and are designated chronic infectious diseases. Some infections initiate an intense but unsuccessful reparative response characterized by the production of abundant granulation tissue and are designated chronic infective granulomas.

PROGRESSIVE TISSUE CHANGES

The tissues of the body may respond to irritation, injury, or increased functional demand other than simply by inflammation. This is especially true when chronic irritation or injury is of a mild degree. Reactive changes to this type of injury are characterized by proliferation and/or alteration of specific cells involved in the injury. These changes, because of their proliferative and altruistic character, are designated *progressive tissue changes.* Such tissue changes may precede or accompany inflammation. Progressive tissue changes include hyperplasia, hypertrophy, keratosis, and metaplasia.

Hyperplasia

Hyperplasia is the response of a tissue or organ to increased function and is a physiologic and altruistic process characterized by an increase in the number of cells making up the tissue or organ (Fig. 49). This response may occur in organs, especially in glands, when there is a demand for greater functional activity. It also occurs in the epithelium covering the surface of the body, such as the skin, mucous membrane of the oral cavity, nasal mucosa, and the mucosa of the respiratory and gastrointestinal tracts. Supporting tissue may also increase its functional activity in an attempt to meet functional demands by increasing the number of supporting cells in an area of increased activity. Supporting tissue hyperplasia often accompanies hyperplasia of surface epithelium.

Hyperplasia of organs, especially glands, occurs when there is a demand for increased secretions. It may be a physiologic response, such as occurs in mammary glands during lactation, or it may be an

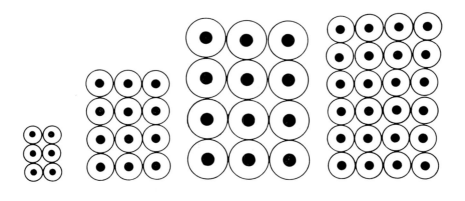

ATROPHY   NORMAL   HYPERTROPHY   HYPERPLASIA

Figure 49. Schematic representation of cell changes in retrogressive and progressive tissue changes.

attempt of glands to meet a deficiency in secretion that has resulted from a loss of tissue owing to disease or injury. Just such a hyperplasia and increase in the size of a gland is exhibited by the parathyroid glands after partial thyroidectomy. The remaining glandular tissue increases in size to a bulk sufficient to compensate for that which was removed. Hyperplasia may also be produced in a gland or tissue to compensate for deficiencies in its functional output. This type of hyperplasia, or enlargement of a gland to compensate for functional deficiency, may be seen in the thyroid glands of puberty age girls whose diets are deficient in iodine. Although growth activity, tissue metabolism, and the demand for thyroid secretion is high at puberty, only a limited quantity of thyroxin is produced by the thyroid because of a low intake of iodine. To compensate, the gland increases the number of cells to produce more thyroid growth hormone; this hyperplasia of thyroid tissue is called a goiter.

Hyperplasia of the tissues of the body surface is usually a response to the demand of these tissues for increased protection against surface irritation. It is demonstrated in the skin in areas of pressure and functional irritation, such as occurs on the hands or fingers when an object such as a golf club, shovel, or periodontal instrument is held tightly. Under the areas of pressure and friction, the epithelium thickens, and the resulting lesion is designated a *callus*. This lesion may be produced in the feet by improperly fitting shoes. Hyperplasia of the gingival tissue may occur from wearing ill-fitting dentures (Fig. 50). As the dentures move, the tissue is rubbed and compressed which results in an increase in thickness of the epithelium to protect against injury (Fig. 51). The underlying connective tissue is also stimulated to proliferate, which results in an in-

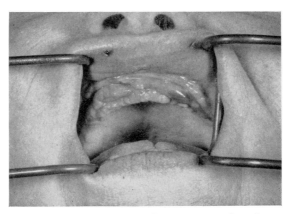

Figure 50. *Hyperplasia*. Gingival hyperplasia associated with wearing ill-fitting dentures.

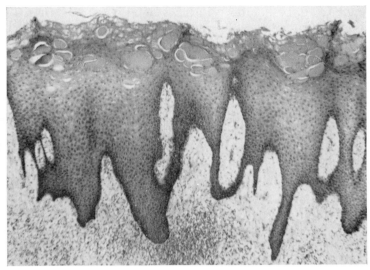

Figure 51. Hyperplasia of surface epithelium with branching and fusing of rete ridges. The epithelium at the surface shows exaggerated formation and retention of intraepithelial hyalin.

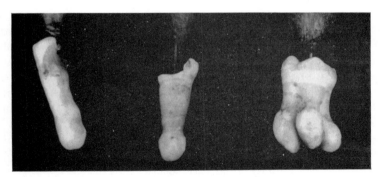

Figure 52. *Hypercementosis.* Apical deposition of cementum in response to increased functional demand.

crease in bulk. Thus the increase in size of the gingiva related to the ill-fitting denture is due to an increase in quantity of both epithelium and connective tissue. An increase in size of the gingiva may be due to other sources of irritation and is discussed in Chapter 11 under gingival disease, page 231.

Hypercementosis occurs on teeth which are in heavy function or about the roots in areas of chronic inflammation. The response to heavy use or inflammation stimulates an excessive deposition of cementum about the apical one-third or one-half of the root (Fig. 52).

This increase in cementum produces a bulbous appearance to the root. The enlargement of the root end makes extraction difficult because the root end is larger than the alveolus through which it must be withdrawn.

Hypertrophy

Hypertrophy is the increase in size of a part owing to an increase in the size of the cells which constitute the part (Fig. 49). Because both hyperplasia and hypertrophy imply an increase in size of a tissue or organ, their use is frequently confused. This confusion is especially true in relation to the gingiva.

Hypertrophy like hyperplasia is a response to meet an increased functional demand. It may be commonly exhibited in muscle and usually reflects a physiologic response of the muscular tissues to an increased functional demand. An arm or a leg repeatedly called upon to do more work than its opposite member will be larger than the other arm or leg owing to an increase in size of the muscle fibers of the extremity doing the greater amount of work, viz., a blacksmith's arm. Observable differences in arm size may be apparent between the right and left arm of normal individuals owing to right- or left-handedness. Pronounced hypertrophy of the muscles of one extremity may be seen when it becomes necessary to compensate for inactivity or paralysis of the other extremity, viz., paralysis of a leg from poliomyelitis. An increase in the size of the uterus to accommodate a developing fetus is due to an increase in the size of the muscle fibers as well as an increase in the number of cells. The individual muscle fibers of the uterus may increase as many as 40 times in order to meet the functional demands of pregnancy. Although smooth musculature (involuntary muscle) does not normally produce new cells or inhibit hyperplasia, the pregnant uterus is an exception.

In the oral region, hypertrophy of the tongue may occur in an individual who has the habit of pushing the tongue against the teeth. Hypertrophy per se occurs only in those tissues or cells with limited ability to reproduce themselves and therefore can only be demonstrated orally in such structures as the tongue and muscles of mastication. Thus, gingival enlargement or hyperplasia should not be misconstrued as gingival hypertrophy.

Hyperkeratosis

Hyperkeratosis is a change occurring in squamous epithelium in response to frictional, chemical, thermal, and sometimes bacterial irritation. It is an attempt by the body to protect the tissue beneath an area of irritation by changing the character of the surface. To fully understand this protective mechanism, it is advisable to discuss briefly the physiology of squamous epithelium. The hard palate and the gingiva are the only areas of the oral mucosa which normally exhibit any degree of protective keratinization.

The layer of epithelial cells immediately in contact with connective tissue is called the basal layer or stratum germinativum (Fig. 53). The cells of this layer have the ability to undergo cell division; this they do continuously at a slow rate unless stimulated by irritation or injury to increase the rate of new cells being formed. As new cells are formed and move toward the surface, changes in morphology occur; they become larger, polyhedral, and develop small projections (spinous process) which unite them with adjacent cells. At this stage of maturation, the cells form a layer called the prickle cell layer or stratum spinosum, which may be several cells in thickness (Fig. 53). As the cells move toward the surface, they become

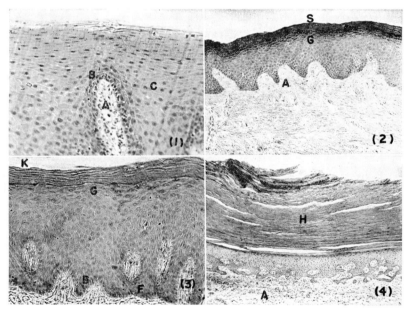

Figure 53. *Epithelial response to irritation.* (1) Nonkeratinized mucosa; connective tissue papillae (A), basal cells (B), stratum spinosum (C) with wide intercellular spaces. (2) Skin; stratum cornium (S), stratum granulosum (G), lamina propria (A). (3) Gingival mucosa showing protective keratinization and hyperplasia; thickened keratin layer (K), increased granular layer (G), increased basal cell proliferation (B), fusion of rete pegs (F). (4) Focal hyperkeratosis of buccal mucosa; heavy production of keratin (H), atrophic epithelium (A).

more removed from the underlying connective tissue from which they obtain nutritional materials needed for metabolism. Cells of the prickle cell layer farthest away from the connective tissue are deprived of adequate nutrition and undergo some degeneration. At this time the cell membrane thickens, the spinous processes disappear, and the amount of cytoplasm increases. At this point maturation may be directed toward the formation of protective keratinization in response to surface stimuli, as in the hard palate and gingiva, or toward nonkeratinization and desquamation, as in the normal buccal mucosa. (The process of keratinization may be initiated in the buccal mucosa in response to surface irritation as a protective measure.) If maturation is directed toward keratinization, the intracellular hyalin increases in quantity. All the squamous cells, at this point of maturation, contain increased amounts of hyalin. In the skin, with the loss of the spiny process of the prickle cell layer, a somewhat translucent layer is present called the stratum lucidum. This layer may be several cells in thickness in the skin but is absent in the oral mucosa. The cells containing intracellular hyalin undergo further degeneration or maturation as evidenced by fragmentation of the nucleus (karyorrhexis), dissemination of chromatin particles throughout the cell, loss of distinctness of the cell boundary or membrane, and the increased compactness of the cytoplasm. Cells showing these characteristics of degeneration comprise the granular layer or stratum granulosum. This layer is not well defined in the oral mucosa, except in areas of protective keratinization or hyperkeratinization (Fig. 53). The outer cells of this layer then lose their cell boundaries, the nuclear fragments disappear, and the cells become flat flakes of keratin on the surface of the skin. This outer layer is the stratum cornium. The small flakes of keratin gradually separate from the surface and fall away (desquamation). This continuing formation, degeneration, and loss of epithelial cells is a slow but constant process which provides a constantly changing covering for the body.

Irritation to the body surface acts as a stimulation for an increased production of new epithelial cells; this activity results in a thicker layer of keratin on the surface of the body. In some areas of the body's surface, the keratin layer is normally very thin or absent, but owing to an increase in the rate of proliferation and degeneration of the squamous epithelium, an accumulation of keratin may occur. This increase in the thickness of keratin on a naturally keratinized surface, or the appearance of keratin on a surface which does not normally become keratinized, is called hyperkeratosis (Fig. 54). The increased production of epithelial cells and the resultant thickening of the keratin layer provide a harder and more protective

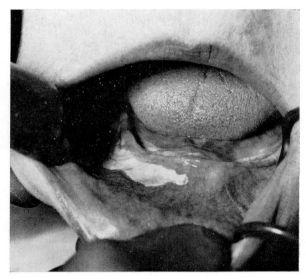

Figure 54. *Hyperkeratosis*. Large white patch of hyperkeratosis of the gingival and alveolar mucosa due to denture irritation.

surface against injury. Hyperkeratosis may or may not accompany hyperplasia. In a *callus* both hyperplasia and hyperkeratosis are present. Hyperkeratosis of the oral mucosa may or may not be associated with hyperplasia. A localized increase in keratin on the oral mucosa gives a white or grayish appearance to the mucosa and is called focal hyperkeratosis.

Focal hyperkeratosis occurs when the tissue is irritated by rough, sharp, or irregular teeth, by poorly fitting dental appliances, or habitual chewing of the lips and cheeks. It is also produced by chemical and thermal irritation associated with heavy smoking of tobacco or the use of highly seasoned foods (Fig. 147). The protective process of keratinization is a physiologic one, but under some situations it does not follow the normal pattern of epithelial maturation but becomes altered so it is no longer beneficial. Such a nonbeneficial alteration then becomes a part of an abnormal process called leukoplakia.

Metaplasia

Metaplasia is a tissue reaction to injury in which the epithelium or connective tissue is transformed into epithelium or connective tissue of another type of lower order (Fig. 55). An example of metaplasia is the transformation of respiratory epithelium to stratified squamous epithelium. The respiratory epithelium is composed

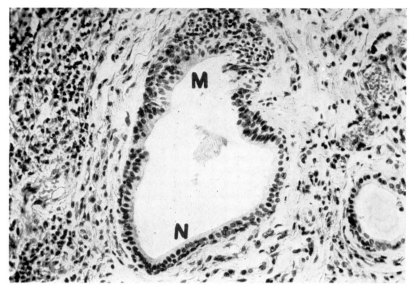

Figure 55. *Metaplasia* of accessory salivary gland duct. Normal ductal epithelium (N), metaplasia of columnar epithelium to squamous type
(M).

of more highly differentiated cells which are less resistant to injury
than the less differentiated squamous epithelium. For example,
chronic irritation of the columnar epithelium of the respiratory
passages of the lungs and the excretory ducts of the salivary glands
may result in the replacement of the columnar epithelium by squamous epithelium. Squamous epithelium is less highly specialized
than columnar epithelium (ductal and respiratory epithelium).
Squamous epithelium has a greater protective ability than columnar
epithelium; therefore, the conversion of columnar epithelium to a
less specialized squamous type of epithelium is a protective reaction
of the tissues.

Metaplasia of mesenchymal connective tissue may occur to form
more highly specialized tissues such as cartilage or bone. This cellular change occurs in response to minor repeated injury or altered
functional demands upon the tissue. This condition is seen in the
tonsil in response to chronic tonsillitis. It is also seen in the gingiva
in response to chronic irritation that is focal in character and produces a local lesion designated an ossifying fibroid epulis.

BLASTOMATOID PROCESSES

Blastomatoid lesions are progressive proliferations in response to
injury. Every act of injury incites a process of repair in which

various types of cells play a part. The proliferative activity of the various tissue elements is normally in a definite physiologic proportion producing an altruistic repair with just the right amount of tissue produced to eliminate the defect. In some processes of repair there is an overzealous proliferation of one tissue element resulting in an exuberant process of repair. Progressive proliferation beyond the normal limits of repair results in the development of tumor-like configurations, which are progressive and permanent in nature. Because the lesion is characterized by proliferation which progresses beyond the normal demand and results in tumescences, it exhibits some of the tendencies of neoplasia. However, these lesions are not autonomous nor are they capable of unlimited growth and cannot be considered as neoplasms (cancer or tumor). Because these lesions have some of the features of neoplasia but are only exaggerated progressive changes, they are called blastomatoid (*blastoma*—neoplasm; *oid*—like) processes.

Blastomatoid lesions are common in the oral cavity because of the frequency with which the oral tissues are injured. They have characteristic features in specific locations. The blastomatoid lesions seen in the oral cavity are listed in the table below.

Blastomatoid Lesions

Granuloma pyogenicum
Traumatic fibroma
Fibroid epulis
Ossifying fibroid epulis
Peripheral giant cell reparative granuloma
Central giant cell reparative granuloma
Tori—palatinus, mandibularis, exostosis
Amputation neuroma
Traumatic hemangioma

Granuloma pyogenicum is a distinct clinical entity which occurs as a sudden exuberant growth of highly vascular granulation tissue (Fig. 56A, B). The exuberant response is due to the intense endothelial proliferation which produces numerous vascular structures of variable size and shape. The vascularity imparts a red or bluish color and a soft consistency to the lesion. The proliferation occurs in the area of surface injury and results in a nodular, usually pedunculated, lesion ranging in size from a few millimeters to a centimeter or more. The lesion may occur suddenly and grow rapidly to a certain size, and then remain static for an indefinite period. The surface is frequently ulcerated and covered with a fibrin membrane through which the dilated vascular spaces appear as red dots. In areas where the adjacent tissue places pressure on the lesion, it be-

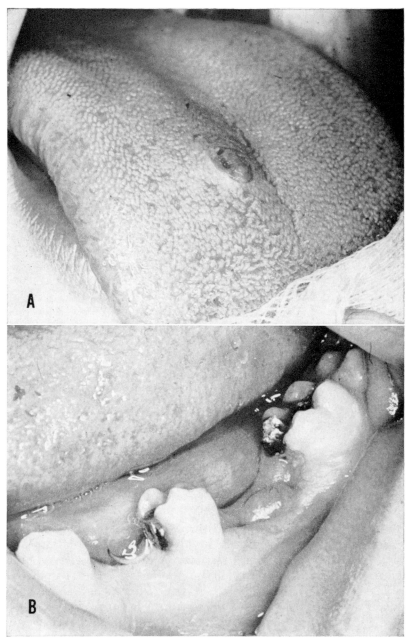

Figure 56. *Granuloma pyogenicum*. A, This is an early lesion with the granulation tissue herniating through a distinct circular defect in the mucosa. The border of the lesion is elevated and rolled. The ulcerated surface is free of fibrinous membrane which is present on the surface of most ulcers. B, The smooth, red, sharply defined nodule protruding from the extraction defect is a mass of granulation tissue. This granulomatous response occurs about bony sequestra.

comes flat and leaf-like and conforms to the available space. The lesion has a tendency to bleed on manipulation.

The lesions occur chiefly on the mucous membrane and skin in areas most subject to injury. The majority of the lesions appear on the hands and the mucous membrane in the oral cavity. The most common sites in the oral cavity are gingiva, tongue, and lip in the order named. The gingival lesions arise from the sulcus of the marginal or papillary gingiva and protrude between the teeth. When they start in the embrasure, they may protrude from both buccal and lingual surfaces and are contoured by the adjacent tissue and teeth. When small, the lesions on the tongue and lip are slightly elevated with an ulcerated summit, but as they increase in size they become pedunculated.

Pregnancy tumor, or granuloma gravidarum, is a granuloma pyogenicum arising from the gingival tissue of a patient who is pregnant (Fig. 57). Because the lesion receives hormonal stimulation during pregnancy, it may grow more rapidly during this period and may regress when the hormonal stimulation is reduced with the termination of the pregnancy. It is associated with pregnancy gingivitis that is discussed in the chapter on gingival disease.

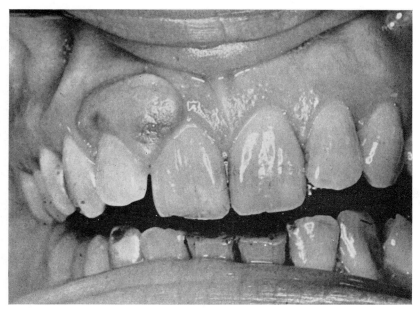

Figure 57. *Granuloma gravidarum.* This soft red pedunculated mass arising from the interdental and subgingival area is flattened and ulcerated by the pressure of the lip. This lesion demonstrated a rapid increase in size during the third month of pregnancy.

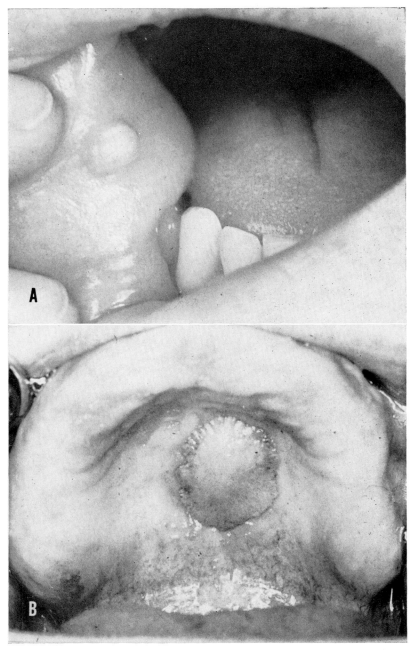

Figure 58. *Traumatic fibroma.* A, The elevated smooth nodule, which is broadest at its base, lighter in color, and firmer than the surrounding mucosa, is typical of this trauma-induced lesion. B, The leaf-like mass attached to the palate by a slender stalk is flattened by the pressure from a denture. The lesion is firm and pale except at the crenated border, which shows a mild inflammatory response. These lesions are often associated with a relief chamber in the denture.

Traumatic fibroma is a slightly elevated nodule of dense scar which is pale, smooth, and firm and varies in size from 3 to 9 millimeters (Fig. 58A, B). The lesion occurs in the buccal mucosa, the lateral border of the tongue, the lip, and the palate in the order named. The lesion is due to an exuberant production of scar in the repair of a small perforating or crushing wound produced by biting or by impingement of tissue against teeth. In very rare cases it results from the spontaneous healing of a granuloma pyogenicum. Because the lesion is asymptomatic and of very limited size, it is not recognized or treated, and therefore the history indicates it was present for a long time.

Fibroid epulis results from the excessive proliferation of fibrous

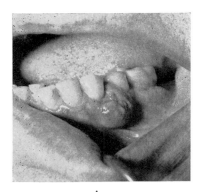

A

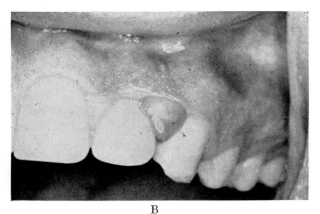

B

Figure 59. *Fibroid epulis.* A, Focal gingival hyperplasia resulting from irritation in gingival sulcus. B, The triangular lesion in the interdental area is the result of proliferation of epithelium and connective tissue due to irritation in the gingival sulcus. The lesion is intensified in color and slightly softer than the normal gingiva.

connective tissue of mature character in response to gingival injury or irritation. Subgingival calculus or a foreign body in the gingival sulcus is the most frequent source of irritation. The origin of the lesion from the gingival sulcus results in a nodular lesion below the gingival margin or interdental papillae (Fig. 59A, B). The lesion is firm and covered by normal gingival mucosa so there is little alteration in color. The lesions are asymptomatic and may be present for a long time. When the lesion arises from the labial gingiva of the lower incisors or the palatal gingiva of the maxillary incisors, it may be impinged between the teeth in occlusion and cause movement of the teeth. Lesions arising in the embrasure usually do not produce separation of the teeth.

Ossifying fibroid epulis (Fig. 60A, B) arises from the gingiva in the same area as the fibroid epulis. It appears as a firm, pale nodule with a broad base arising from the marginal or papillary gingiva. It projects more abruptly from the gingiva and is firmer in consistency than the fibroid epulis because the center of the lesion is composed of bone. The bone originates as the result of metaplasia of connective tissue in the center of the lesion or as the result of chronic irritation to periosteum or periodontal membrane, inciting bone formation. The lesions grow slowly without symptoms and rarely exceed a centimeter in size.

Peripheral giant cell reparative granuloma (giant cell epulis) is a tumor of gingiva produced by injury to periodontal membrane or bone, probably with associated hemorrhage and bone resorption (Fig. 61A, B). In the process of osseous repair there is destruction of bone by specialized cells which develop from connective tissue for the specific purpose of resorbing bone. These cells are large multinucleated cells called osteoblasts which characterize this lesion and give it the name of giant cell epulis.

The giant cell lesion arises as a smooth tumescence of gingiva or interdental tissue, but as it increases in size, it may become somewhat lobulated. Since the lesion is highly vascular, it is soft in consistency and intensified in color varying from bright- to bluish-red depending on the state of the vascular supply. The lesion appears suddenly and increases rapidly in size. The surface of the lesion contacted by other tissues usually becomes ulcerated and covered by a heavy yellow fibrinous membrane (Fig. 62). There is a tendency for the lesion to bleed on manipulation, frequently the only symptom presented. The lesion appears fixed to underlying bone.

The histologic features of the lesion are proliferation of fibroblasts and endothelium to produce a highly vascular stroma in which the vascularity is in the form of sinusoids. Occasional inflammatory cells are present and osteoclastic-type giant cells are present in varying

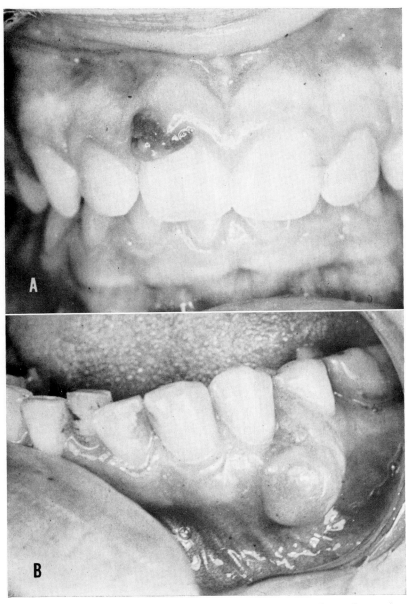

Figure 60. *Ossifying fibroid epulis.* A, This lesion arising from the marginal gingiva is due to injury of the alveolar crest. Granulation tissue shows metaplasia to bone arising from the periodontal membrane of the alveolar crest due to subgingival trauma. This is an early fibro-osseous lesion. B, This hard nodular mass having the same color as the surrounding gingiva is attached by a small stalk to the attached gingiva. The lesion is composed of fibrous tissue with central ossification arising as the result of injury to the periosteum.

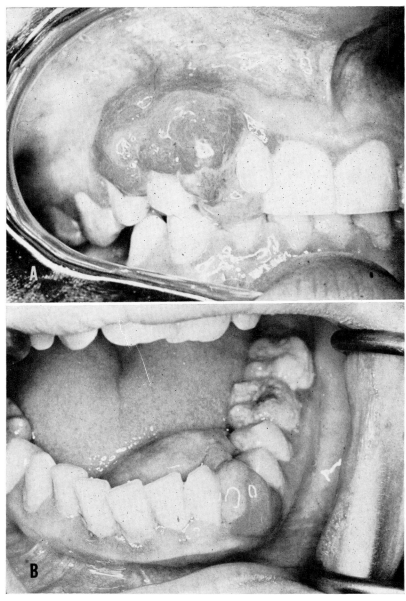

Figure 61. *Peripheral giant cell reparative granuloma.* A, This nodular soft red lesion is contoured by the pressure of lip and cheek to fill the canine fossa and the embrasure between the teeth. B, This lesion arising from the embrasure and extending slightly to the buccal and extensively to the lingual has been present for nine months. The lesion is soft and has been molded by the pressure of the lips and tongue. The lesion is intensely red and the sublingual portion shows surface ulceration.

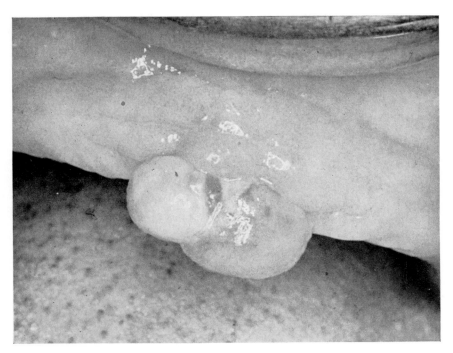

Figure 62. *Peripheral giant cell reparative granuloma.* The nodular, slightly
     pedunculated lesion of the edentulous ridge was initiated by trauma
     from the patient's denture. The white portion of the lesion is ulcer-
     ated and surfaced by a fibrin membrane.

numbers. They are usually in focal zones scattered throughout the
vascular stroma. The lesion contains varying quantities of phagocytized hemosiderin at the site of origin as well as a zone of productive
osteitis. The presence of the osteoclastic-type cell associated with
the evidence of hemorrhage and bone repair is an indication of the
etiology of the lesion. The exuberant production of the osteoclasts
is evidence of the overzealous repair which places the lesion in this
group of blastomatoid lesions.

Because of the deep seat of origin of the lesion, the reparative
granuloma is frequently incompletely removed and rapidly recurs.
The recurrence may be so rapid as to be alarming to both patient
and surgeon. However, with total removal the lesion is cured by
local excision.

Central giant cell reparative granuloma (central giant cell tumor)
also is a lesion associated with the overzealous repair in bone (Fig.
63). The lesion arises from the center of the bone rather than from
its surface. The peripheral lesion arises from the periosteum; the

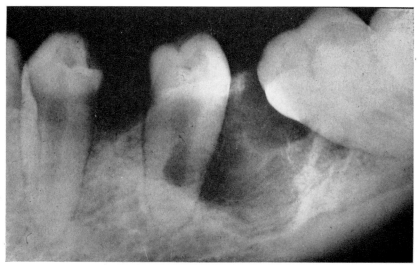

Figure 63. *Central giant cell reparative granuloma.* The lobulated area of radiolucency has a sharp arcuate border and is partitioned by delicate trabeculae giving it a multilocular or "soap bubble" appearance.

medullary (central) lesion arises from the endosteum. Like the peripheral lesion it is characterized by proliferation of connective tissue and endothelium to produce a granulomatous tissue with varying numbers of giant cells. The phagocytized hemosiderin and the productive osteitis are also a characteristic feature of the lesion. All of the changes present indicate the reactive nature of the lesion. Microscopically, the peripheral and central lesions are identical. The central lesion probably arises as the result of trauma with intraosseous hemorrhage which causes bone destruction and initiates the repair which becomes excessive and initiates further destruction of bone.

The lesion is noted clinically because of expansion of the buccal plates and occasional looseness of the teeth. Radiographic examination demonstrates a multiloculated cyst-like lesion of the jaw with some resorption of roots that project into the radiolucent area. The lesions are slowly progressive and may reach large size, producing considerable facial deformity. Surgical treatment is indicated, and like peripheral lesions, it must be total to be curative and without recurrence. Recurrence is frequent because of incomplete removal.

Recurrence of either the peripheral or central lesion may be indicative of initiation by hyperparathyroidism (p. 273). In the patient with a parathyroid adenoma, there is an overproduction of parathyroidin which mobilizes calcium from the bones. This usually results in the production of fibrocystic lesions in bone, but in a few instances, the same type of overzealous repair initiated by trauma occurs and the lesion is identical with the giant cell reparative granuloma. The hemosiderin imparts a brown color to the lesion, therefore, the lesion is designated "brown tumor" of hyperpara-

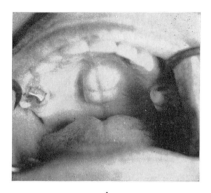

A

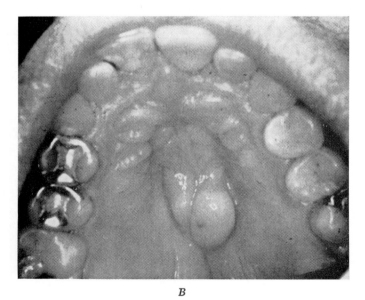

B

Figure 64. *Torus palatinus.* A, A blastomatoid change characterized by an increased production of bone along palatal suture. B, The irregular nodular mass in the midline of the palate has a small ulcer at the summit of the larger mass. The very thin mucosa over the nodule of bone is subject to frequent trauma and ulceration.

thyroidism. This endocrine-produced lesion is not cured by surgery and recurrence is the rule. Therefore, when a giant cell lesion recurs, there is always a suggestion of its being induced by parathyroid dysfunction, and clinical laboratory procedures are indicated to rule out the presence of a "brown tumor" of hyperparathyroidism. The procedures include the evaluation of the serum calcium and alkaline phosphatase values both of which will be elevated in hyperparathyroidism.

Torus palatinus is a hard bony lesion arising in the midline of the palate (Fig. 64A, B). It may arise in any part of the midpalatal suture as a smooth or lobulated hard lesion covered by normal mucosa. The lesion starts in early life and grows slowly reaching a large size and prevalence by 30 years of age. The etiology is not completely understood but may be a proliferation of osseus tissue along the midpalatal suture in response to heavy occlusal stress. The lesion occurs in about 25 percent of the population. It is two times as common in women as in men. It is frequently traumatized which may cause ulceration.

Torus mandibularis is a nodular growth of osseus tissue on the posterior lingual aspect of the mandible just above the mylohyoid line (Fig. 65). It is usually bilateral and may extend from the cuspid to the distal surface of the last molar as a series of discrete or fused nodules 3 to 6 millimeters in size. In some individuals both palatal and mandibular tori may be present. The tori are of concern to the patient who is a denture candidate. Ulcers frequently occur on the summits of the nodules because the mucosa, which is thin over the bone, is injured by hard foods.

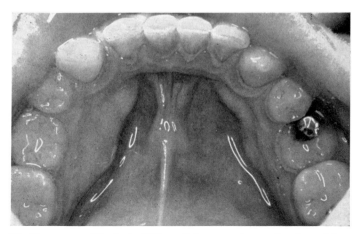

Figure 65. *Torus mandibularis.* Bilateral increase in production of bone above the mylohyoid line. This is a blastomatoid change.

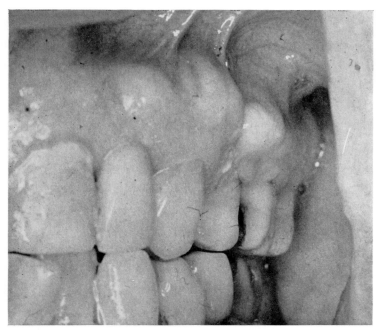

Figure 66. *Exostoses.* These smooth hard nodular excrescences over the buccal aspect of the roots of the teeth result from excess bone production in response to hyperfunction.

Exostosis (Fig. 66) occurs as a nodular bony protuberance on the buccal surfaces of the maxilla and mandible. It may accompany palatal and mandibular tori. In most instances the exostosis occurs over teeth positioned towards the labial with very thin labial bone. Exostoses are usually reactive to heavy functional stress and occur as nodules over teeth in heavy function. When all the teeth are in heavy function, the nodules may fuse together to produce a nodular ledge. Like tori, exostoses may be traumatized with resultant ulceration. The ulcers over exostoses and tori are usually chronic because of periosteal injury resulting in bone necrosis, which necessitates sequestration of the necrotic bone before healing can occur. Exostoses are less common than tori and do not exhibit the same sex preference.

Amputation neuroma is a proliferation of excessive nervous tissue in a zone of repair following the loss of continuity of a nerve owing to trauma. Regeneration of the nerve is attempted but may be prevented by the presence of scar tissue. The nerve continues to proliferate and an excess of nerve tissue develops. When near the surface, the lesion is painful on pressure. Lesions arising from the inferior alveolar nerve due to injury during removal of impacted third molars produce pain in the jaw.

Traumatic hemangiomas are elevated, thin-walled, large vascular spaces in the submucosa which produce surface elevation, are purplish in color, are soft and fluctuant in character, and blanch on prolonged pressure (Fig. 67A). They occur most frequently on the

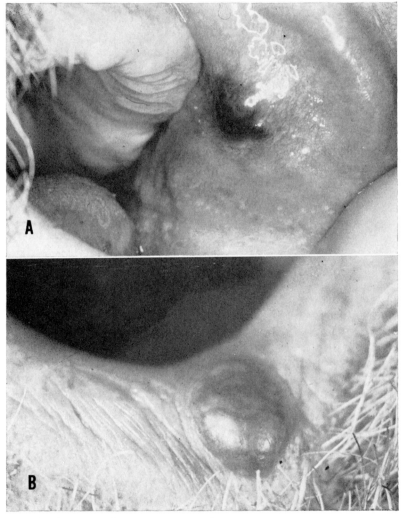

Figure 67. *Traumatic hemangioma.* A, The elevated bluish lesion in the buccal mucosa is soft and blanches on pressure. B, The smooth elevated nodule with a broad base is purplish in color, soft to touch, and blanches with pressure. It is produced by mechanical injury.

lip of older men (Fig. 67B). They are several times more common in men than women and, in both sexes, are more common on the lower lip. They may occur on the tongue, especially the inferior surface or the buccal mucosa. They arise from varicosities, in areas of telangiectasia, and are caused by mechanical injury. In older men who have solar cheilitis, there is terminal dilatation of terminal vessels with weakened walls which dilate and form thin-walled, blood-filled spaces in the upper submucosa. Focal saccular dilatation occurs in varicosities which, if close to the surface, produce the "blood blister" appearance typical of traumatic angiomas. They also occur from perforating wounds which produce an opening in the walls of both artery and vein permitting the shunting of blood from artery directly to vein. The increased pressure in the vein causes saccular dilatation which, if near the surface, produces the typical picture of the angioma. They are also called arteriovenous aneurysms.

BIBLIOGRAPHY

Ake, N., and Landt, H.: Hyperplasia of the oral tissues in denture cases. Acta Odont. Scand., 27:481, 1969.

Anderson, J. R.: Auto-antibodies in the diseases of man. Brit. Med. Bull., 19: 251, 1963.

Black, M. M., and Wagner, B. M.: Dynamic Pathology. St. Louis, C. V. Mosby Co., 1964.

Bostick, W. L.: The vascular-cellular dynamics of inflammation. Oral Surg., 2:425, 1949.

Dunphy, J. E., and Udupa, K. N.: Chemical and histochemical sequences in the normal healing of wounds. New Eng. J. Med., 253:847, 1955.

Editorial: Reticuloendothelial function. J.A.M.A., 199:419, 1967.

Holborow, E. J., Ed.: Antibodies. Brit. Med. Bull., 19:169, 1963.

Menkin, V.: Dynamics of Inflammation. New York, The Macmillan Co., 1940.

Ranney, R. R., and Zander, H. A.: Allergic periodontal disease in sensitized squirrel monkeys. J. Periodont., 41:12, 1970.

Resistance to Infection. Therap. Notes, 73:8, 1966.

Rizzo, A. A., and Mergenhagen, S. E.: Studies on the significance of hypersensitivity in periodontal disease. Periodontics, 3:271, 1965.

Robbins, S. L.: Pathology, 3rd ed. Philadelphia, W. B. Saunders Co., 1967.

Wissler, R. W., Fitch, F. W., and Lavia, M. F.: The reticuloendothelial system in antibody formation. Ann. N. Y. Acad. Sci., 88:134, 1960.

Wound healing. Therap. Notes, 71:68, 1964.

Chapter 5

NEOPLASIA

DEFINITION

The term neoplasia refers to that formation of abnormal new tissue occurring when the normal regulative processes of cellular differentiation and proliferation have been lost. The subject of neoplasia is a complex but interesting and important one because of the frequency with which neoplastic disease occurs in the population. The lesion that develops in neoplasia is technically called a neoplasm, although the terms *tumor* and *cancer* are used extensively, especially by the laity.

The process of neoplasia is one that takes place within body cells causing them to undergo spontaneous, independent, uncontrolled, and unlimited growth. Without apparent reason, cells responsible for forming mature, functioning tissue lose their normal processes of differentiation and proliferation. They then produce new cells which are quantitatively and qualitatively abnormal and replace the tissue in which the neoplastic process occurs. The area of origin of a neoplasm may be very small but may rapidly increase in size to involve an entire organ or part. The neoplasm may remain confined to the site of origin or it may extend to other areas of the body. In many instances neoplasms spread into or replace vital areas and cause the death of the host.

EPIDEMIOLOGY

Neoplastic disease occurs in a large part of the animal kingdom; in humans it involves both sexes of all ages, although it is most common in the older age group. Because there is a high incidence of neoplasms in patients over 50 years of age, this age is sometimes called the "cancer age." Some races show greater tendency for cancer of specific areas than other races. Furthermore, one sex may have a greater incidence of cancer of specific organs than the other sex. The accompanying charts demonstrate the areas of the body most frequently involved and the incidence of cancer and death according to sex and anatomic location.

INCIDENCE OF CANCER AND DEATH
(According to Site and Sex)

Site of Origin	% Incidence of Cancer		% Deaths Due to Cancer	
	Male	Female	Male	Female
Mouth	6.2	2.9	3.3	1.1
Respiratory	12.3	2.5	21.6	4.0
Digestive	33.0	23.3	35.0	33.5
Genital	10.8	24.4	11.2	19.9
Urinary	7.0	3.4	6.0	3.5
Leukemia and Lymphoma	6.3	4.0	10.5	8.6

INCIDENCE OF CANCER IN VARIOUS ANATOMIC SITES

Site	Peak Incidence (Years of Age)
Kidney	0–4
Bone	15–25
Brain	40–45
Skin	60–65
Abdominal organs	60–65
Digestive tract	60–80

In the past 50 years the incidence of neoplastic disease has shown a progressive increase which is in part an actual and in part an apparent increase. During this period cancer has risen from tenth place to second as a cause of death. The *actual* increase in incidence is due to technologic advances (new chemicals, radiation, and other factors) and to our mode of living, which makes it possible to come into contact with carcinogenic agents. For example, with the marked increase in cigarette smoking, there has been an alarming increase in cancer of the lungs owing to inhalation of the combustion products of tobacco. The *apparent* increase in neoplastic disease is due to public health measures which have increased the life expectancy to above 60 years, so that more people are living to the "cancer age." Because cancer affects all ages of both sexes and stands second as a cause of death, it presents one of our most perplexing health problems.

ETIOLOGY

The cause of neoplasia is unknown. Why a particular cell or group of cells spontaneously undergo unlimited, progressive, independent growth is a perplexing problem which as yet has defied intensive research. However, there are many things known about some of the factors predisposing or influencing the development of neoplasia. These factors are discussed here as hereditary, extrinsic, and developmental factors.

Hereditary Factors

There is considerable evidence that heredity plays a significant role in the development of neoplastic disease. Although neoplasia is not generally considered to be an inheritable disease, some factors of susceptibility or immunity appear to be present. The influence of heredity has been demonstrated in mice; some strains have been developed that are almost 100 percent susceptible to certain neoplasms and other strains have been bred that are cancer-resistant. In humans the importance of heredity can be demonstrated by the frequency with which identical twins develop identical neoplasms at about the same age even though their environments may have been different. It is also significant that some individuals develop more than one type of neoplasm. There are families in which nearly all members develop neoplasms of the same organ at about the same age. This age is some ten or more years younger than the average age for such a neoplasm of the same organ in the population at large. Although the familial occurrence of neoplasia is rare, retinoblastoma is a good example of a neoplasm having a familial pattern. There is also a familial tendency for multiple polyposis which almost invariably leads to carcinoma. All of these and many more observations indicate that heredity plays an important part in susceptibility to neoplastic disease.

Extrinsic Factors

Extrinsic factors are environmental in nature, numerous, and important to the development of neoplastic disease. Examples of various environmental factors will serve to indicate their nature, wide variety, and importance.

MECHANICAL IRRITATION. Clinical observations suggest that chronic mechanical irritation serves as a causal factor in cancer, viz., the development of cancer associated with wearing loose or ill-fitting dentures. Hyperplasia occurs in response to irritation, but, in some instances, the new cells become neoplastic and produce a neoplasm of the alveolar ridge. The new cells in hyperplasia cause an increase in the bulk of tissue, but they duplicate the picture of normal cells. The new cells in an area of cancer may resemble the normal cells but do not duplicate them, and they proliferate rapidly even though the irritation is removed.

CHEMICALS. Neoplastic causal factors can be demonstrated in a large variety of chemical substances. The first experimental production of a neoplasm in a laboratory was produced by rubbing coal tar

9

on the ear of a rabbit. Today, in high-cancer strains of laboratory animals, neoplasms can be produced by many substances refined from coal tar. These chemicals and many others that influence the development of cancer are called *carcinogens.* Some of the hormones and other substances produced by the body have a carcinogenic effect as well as a variety of other chemicals, notably arsenic. Hormonal factors are important in the development of cancers of the breast, uterus, and prostate. The most common tumor of the young female breast is hormonally induced through the effect of repeated cyclic stimulation by ovarian hormones. Cancers of the uterus and breast are also associated with estrogenic stimulation, and, because of the intense effect produced by the sex hormones, they are used in some phases of the treatment of cancers of the breast, uterus, and prostate.

IRRADIATION. Irradiation by x rays, radioactive material, and sunlight all play an important part in the production of cancer. X-ray irradiation in a single massive dose or in repeated small doses predisposes the skin to the development of cancer. This is evidenced by the frequency with which dentists and technicians develop cancer of the hands from habitually holding x-ray films in patients' mouths for exposure. The repeated small quantity of x ray received is cumulative, and after a period of years the individual develops an x-ray dermatitis which progresses to cancer (Fig. 68). With massive doses of x ray producing tissue destruction (the so-called x-ray burn), healing is delayed sometimes for years, and cancer develops at the site of attempted repair.

Small doses of radioactive material ingested or introduced into the body may also produce cancer; this occurred in watch-dial

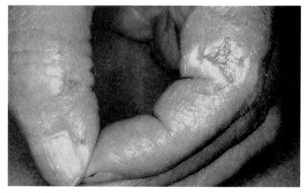

Figure 68. *X-ray dermatitis.* X-ray burns on thumb and forefinger from frequently holding x-ray films in patients' mouths. Squamous cell carcinoma (skin cancer) often develops in these areas.

painters in the 1920's. In making luminous watch dials, women employees applied radioactive paint with a fine brush which they pointed with their lips. Unfortunately, by this maneuver, small quantities of radioactive material in the form of radium salts were ingested. The radium salts united with calcium and became stored in the bones. After less than a year of this practice, nearly all of the women developed cancer of the bone.

SUNLIGHT. Sunlight is a potent factor in producing cancer of the skin, especially in individuals who have little natural pigment for protection. Over a period of years, repeated exposure conditions the skin so that later in life numerous small skin cancers may develop on the face or other exposed parts. The face is the most common site and the cancers are of a specific type—basal cell carcinoma.

There also is a definite relationship between cancer of the lip and exposure to sunlight. Individuals, usually males who have light skin and spend much time out of doors, develop solar cheilitis which predisposes to cancer of the lip. Solar cheilitis can be easily recognized when viewing the lips and should be called to the attention of the patient. The lip changes in solar cheilitis occur slowly over a period of years and, therefore, present a varying appearance, depending upon the degree of advancement. The first change is the loss of vertical fissures of the lower lip owing to atrophy of the epithelium, which also produces a smooth shiny parchment-like quality to the epithelium of the exposed vermilion border. As the process progresses, the epithelium shows increased cornification and imparts a bluish-gray opacity to the lip. In limited areas small whitish plaques may develop. There is a tendency for small flakes of keratin to occur on the surface along with small cracks or ulcers (Fig. 69). In the more advanced stages periodic ulceration occurs, especially with continued exposure to sunlight. In the advanced condition, the lip is smooth, grayish white, or mottled bluish gray with flaking and periodic superficial ulceration. Such changes predispose to

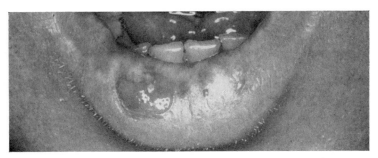

Figure 69. *Solar cheilitis.* The vermilion border is thin, smooth, opaque, and ulcerated from prolonged exposure to sun and wind.

cancer of the lip. However, if the predisposing changes are recognized early, the patient can prevent cancer by protecting his lips from exposure to sunlight. It should be the duty of all who treat the mouth and inspect the lips to recognize the lip changes noted above and to advise the patient of their significance.

Other extrinsic factors such as age, race, socioeconomic status, occupation, and habits are related to the development of cancer, but the association is not as direct as the factors discussed above and, therefore, will not be elaborated upon.

Developmental Factors

Developmental factors are inherent forces of growth and differentiation responsible for the proper development of a tissue or organ. These forces may be disturbed during the development of a tissue or part so that the cells lose their ability to continue differentiation while at the same time they retain or accentuate their growth potential. When a developing tissue undergoes independent proliferation at some stage of differentiation short of final maturity, a neoplasm is produced. An excellent example of a developmental neoplasm is the ameloblastoma arising from the developing enamel organ. Disturbances of development may play a part in a variety of neoplasms, but the mechanism is not well understood.

GENERAL CHARACTERISTICS

Neoplasia occur in any tissue of the body and exhibit a variety of characteristics distinctive for each neoplasm in each type of tissue. For this reason it is necessary to describe and to label each type of neoplasm so that it can be distinguished and placed in its proper position in the large field of neoplasia. Two large divisions of neoplasms are designated—*benign* and *malignant*.

Benign Neoplasms

The benign neoplasm arises in any area of the body from any type of tissue and presents specific features which give it a somewhat predictable behavior. The benign neoplasm generally grows slowly because of a limited ability for proliferation, but it has a high degree of ability for differentiation. The cells making up a benign neoplasm duplicate well the parent type of cell and resemble normal cells. Cells of a benign neoplasm have a level of differentiation high enough in some instances to retain normal but independent functional activity. Benign neoplastic cells divide with a nearly typical mitotic pattern resulting in an expansile lesion which does not invade other tissues but does produce pressure atrophy of surrounding tissue as its bulk slowly increases (Fig. 70). With

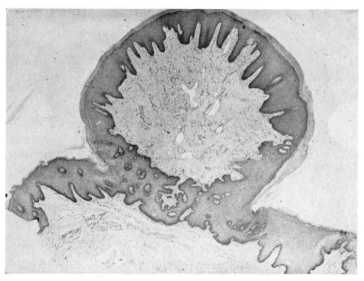

Figure 70. *Fibroepithelial papilloma.* A benign lesion of papillomatous character demonstrating expansile growth.

expansile growth there frequently is compression of the stroma surrounding the developing mass giving the neoplasm the appearance of being surrounded by a fibrous capsule. Because of its slow growth, high level of differentiation, limited ability to invade, and somewhat limited potential for growth, the benign neoplasm is of local significance and can be totally removed by surgery and a cure accomplished. These factors are characteristic of a benign neoplasm and for that reason it is referred to as a tumor by the lay person. The word tumor probably has no place in a scientific classification of neoplasms, but it does have an important role to play in describing, to a patient, the nature of his neoplasm. When a person is told he has a tumor, it indicates to him that he has a growth of tissue limited to one small area of his body which can be removed by surgery and a cure affected.

Malignant Neoplasms

In contrast to the benign neoplasm is the malignant neoplasm. The malignant neoplasm also arises from any type of tissue in any part of the body, but it exhibits a rapid rate of proliferation and a poor level of differentiation (so poor that it may be impossible to recognize the type of tissue from which the neoplasm arises). Because of rapid growth and poor differentiation, malignant cells develop bizarre mitotic figures and grow by infiltration rather than expansion. In infiltrative growth the surrounding tissue is replaced completely and no distinct boundaries or capsule develops (Fig. 71). Absence of a tissue boundary and extension by growth between various tissue structures result in widespread and extensive invasion resulting in difficulty of localization and removal. The invasion occurs in any area, often in vascular channels. When vascular spaces are invaded, the invading cells find a favorable habitat for growth, and they proliferate extensively within the lumen of a blood vessel or lymphatic. The loosely arranged new cells may propagate along the lumens of vessels and spread the neoplasm for some distance; or, they may be broken away from the main mass and be carried by blood or lymph to some distant area where they become lodged and set up a second foci of growth. This discontinuous spread from one area to another is called *metastasis*, a feature of malignant neoplasms. A neoplasm with a low level of differentiation, rapid invasive growth, and discontinuous spread is called a malignant neoplasm and is generally known to the lay person as cancer. Cancer, like tumor, is a term understood by laity and may be used to designate to a patient that he has a malignant neoplasm, but it does not designate the type of neoplasm. Thus, to the patient, the term cancer means that he has a new growth which is difficult to remove,

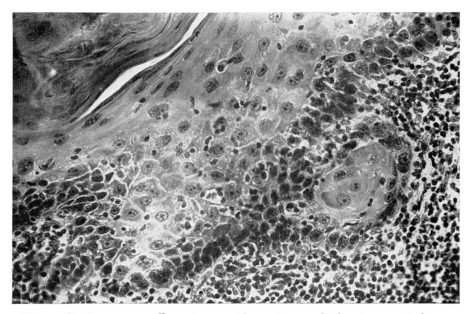

Figure 71. *Squamous cell carcinoma.* Photomicrograph showing atypical proliferation of epithelium with small islands below the basal layer demonstrating invasive growth of a malignant neoplasm.

will spread to other areas of his body, and, if not entirely removed, will continue to grow and ultimately will cause his death.

SUMMARY OF DIFFERENCES BETWEEN BENIGN AND MALIGNANT CANCERS

Characteristics	Benign	Malignant
Metastases	Never	Almost always
Recurrence	Rare	Frequent
Mitosis	Almost normal	Rapid, atypical
Growth	Expansile, slow	Invasive, rapid
Character of cells	Nearly normal	Poorly differentiated
Limitation	Often encapsulated	Not encapsulated

This summary is only general and does not include specific and detailed clinical and microscopic differences, which are necessary to make the diagnosis of a specific neoplasm.

CLASSIFICATION

Neoplasms of both benign and malignant types may arise from either epithelial or connective tissue, or both, and may be named according to the type of tissue from which they originate as well as according to their nature. In some types of mesenchymal neoplasms, two or three varieties of tissue may be present in varying proportions. When more than one type of tissue is present in a neoplasm, it is named according to the behavior and type of tissue which predominates. For example, where two different types of tissue are present, the names of the tissues are combined to form a prefix indicating the types of tissue present. Thus, a tumor composed of fibrous tissue and nerve tissue with the fibrous tissue predominating is called a neurofibroma. The suffix, -oma, is a nonspecific term which usually implies a neoplasm. The term *sarcoma* refers to a malignant neoplasm arising from mesenchymal tissue; however, it should be pointed out that the suffix, -oma, is sometimes used along with the tissue of origin to designate malignant neoplasms of mesenchymal or epithelial origin, viz., lymphoma, endothelioma, epithelioma. If a neoplasm consists of *nervous* tissue and *fibrous* tissue and has malignant characteristics, the ending *sarcoma* is used and the lesion is designated as a neurofibrosarcoma. The term *carcinoma* is used to designate malignant neoplasms of epithelial origin, viz., squamous cell carcinoma. It is important to classify neoplasms according to tissue origin and according to their benign or malignant character because each neoplasm presents a different behavior pattern. Knowledge of the behavior pattern of a neoplasm is essential to direct adequate treatment. The following classification of neoplasms indicates the variety of neoplasms which may occur in the body. It is a simplified classification based upon histogenesis.

CLASSIFICATION OF NEOPLASMS

Origin	Benign	Malignant
Epithelium		
Squamous	Papilloma	Squamous cell carcinoma
		Basal cell carcinoma
Columnar	Adenoma	Adenocarcinoma
	Polyp	
Specialized	Hydatid mole	Choriocarcinoma
	Ameloblastoma	
Mesenchymal Tissue		
Fibrous tissue	Fibroma	Fibrosarcoma
Nervous tissue	Neuroma	Neurosarcoma
	Neurofibroma°	Neurofibrosarcoma°
Myxomatous	Myxoma	Myxosarcoma
	Myxofibroma°	Myxofibrosarcoma°
Adipose	Lipoma	Liposarcoma
Bone	Osteoma	Osteogenic sarcoma
Cartilage	Chondroma	Chondrosarcoma
Blood vessels	Hemangioma	Hemangiosarcoma
Lymph vessels	Lymphangioma	Lymphangiosarcoma
Melanoblasts	Nevus (melanotic)	Malignant melanoma (melanosarcoma)
Hemopoietic, lymphoid and reticuloendothelial tissue		Leukemia
		Lymphoblastoma
		Myeloma
		Reticulum cell sarcoma
Odontogenic tissue	Odontogenic myxoma	
	Odontogenic fibroma	
Mixed		
Odontogenic tissue	Composite odontoma	
Salivary gland tissue	Mixed tumors of salivary glands	Malignant mixed tumors of salivary glands

Note: two or more tissue combinations may occur.

Although incomplete, this classification gives a general idea of the complex nature of the process of neoplasia. Only the common neoplasms occurring in the oral cavity and extra-oral neoplasms of dental significance are discussed in this book.

Neoplasms of Epithelial Origin

Papilloma is a benign neoplasm arising from squamous epithelium and occurring with some frequency in the oral cavity (Fig. 72). It occurs in the gingiva, palate, tongue, floor of mouth, and lip as a lobulated or filiform elevation 2 to 5 millimeters in diameter. It is white and has a firmer consistency than the normal mucosa. Growth

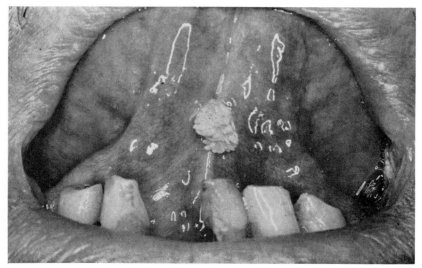

Figure 72. *Papilloma.* The filiform white lesion on the lingual frenum is a papilloma.

is very slow and the lesions rarely reach a centimeter in diameter. Complete surgical removal provides a cure.

Basal cell carcinoma is a neoplasm arising from squamous epithelium which duplicates the pattern of the cells of the basal layer of the epithelium. Basal cell carcinoma occurs most often on the face of older people, especially men who have had prolonged exposure to intense sunlight, or people with light complexions who have little resistance to actinic radiation. There is a positive correlation between exposure to sun and the development of basal cell carcinoma. A basal cell carcinoma may be a flat or slightly elevated lesion 3 to 10 millimeters in size and whitish or reddish pink in color. The center of the lesion may be scaly or ulcerated. The early lesions are usually scaly, whereas the older lesions are ulcerated. As the lesion grows, the border becomes slightly elevated and pearly white, while the ulcerated center becomes larger and deeper. Very advanced lesions may involve an area of several inches. Basal cell carcinoma has a tendency to invade tissue locally but rarely metastasizes. Lesions may be destroyed by x-ray irradiation or removed by surgery. Type of treatment indicated depends on location, size, and changes present in the skin.

Cornifying squamous cell carcinoma (epithelioma) is the most common malignant neoplasm of the oral region. It is most common on the lip but also occurs on the tongue, alveolar ridge, floor of mouth, palate, and in the buccal mucosa. Squamous cell carcinoma occurs predominately on the lower lip of males of advanced age. Carcinoma of the lip may present a variety of appearances depending upon the degree of advancement. The early lesion may be a slightly elevated plaque firmer than the surrounding vermilion and whitish or grayish in color. It may be a keratinized plaque (Fig. 73) or a superficial ulcer (Fig. 74). As the lesion advances it becomes slightly elevated and ulcerated (Fig. 75). The border is rolled and grayish. Large lesions may be either fungating or destructive. Carcinoma of the lip metastasizes late to the regional lymph nodes and, therefore, offers a good prognosis when treated early. Ad-

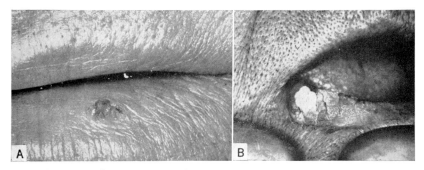

Figure 73. A, *Early squamous cell carcinoma.* Small, slightly elevated hyperkeratotic lesion in the mid-vermilion of the left lip. B, Large hyperkeratotic plaque on lower lip. The heavy white keratotic area at the angle of the mouth showing some "rolling" of the border is carcinomatous. This patient had held a pipe in this area for many years.

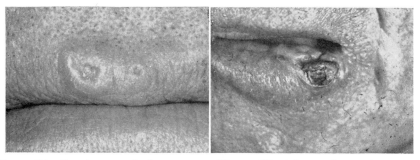

Figure 74. *Carcinoma of the upper lip.* Early cancer showing typically depressed center with a whitish elevated periphery. The depressed center is due to early ulceration.

Figure 75. *Advanced carcinoma of the lip.* Ulcerated lesion with elevation at the border and thickening of the lip. This is characteristic location for lip cancer.

vanced carcinoma of the lip has a guarded prognosis even with extensive treatment. Carcinoma of the lip may be treated with either x-ray irradiation or surgery. Both methods provide a cure and satisfactory cosmetic results.

Carcinoma of the tongue usually starts on the lateral border either as an elevated white lesion or as an ulcer (Fig. 76). It may invade the under surface of the tongue and extend into the floor of the mouth. The patient frequently states that the lesion was initiated by biting his tongue, and the acceptance of this statement causes the true nature of the lesion to be overlooked. In most instances, the patient bit the tongue because the neoplasm was present but had not been recognized. Carcinoma of the tongue metastasizes early. The more posterior the lesion, the poorer the prognosis. Even with radical treatment early carcinoma of the tongue offers a poor prognosis. Carcinoma of the tongue may be treated by surgery or x-ray irradiation, or by surgery with postoperative irradiation.

Carcinoma of the alveolar ridge is usually associated with wearing ill-fitting dentures or with sharp broken teeth which produce chronic irritation of the gingival mucosa. Chewing tobacco or using snuff may be an initiating factor. This variety of carcinoma usually starts as an ulcer, which enlarges and becomes elevated at the periphery, or it may start as an area of hyperkeratinization. Carcinoma of the alveolar ridge metastasizes late, but may still have a poor prognosis because of its proximity to bone which it invades making treatment difficult. Treatment of carcinoma of the alveolar ridge is usually surgical excision and is severely mutilating because of the required

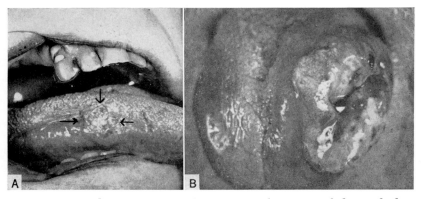

Figure 76. A, *Early carcinoma of the tongue.* The extent of this early lesion is indicated by the arrows. The lesion followed irritation from a broken partial denture clasp. B, *Fungating lesion with central necrosis.* The patient stated this lesion started from biting his tongue.

resection of the jaw. Irradiation is not satisfactory because of the intolerance of bone to x-ray irradiation.

Adenoma and *adenocarcinoma* arise in the oral region from the accessory or major salivary glands, but these neoplasms are not common. Because they arise in the substance of the gland, they are clinically manifest only as swellings in the areas of origin (Fig. 77A, B). The most common neoplasms of the salivary glands are the mixed salivary gland tumors which, as the name indicates, are both epithelial and mesenchymal in origin. Epithelial and stromal elements proliferate in varying proportions to produce the neoplasm. These neoplasms present a wide variety of combinations of epithelial and mesenchymal elements which determine their behavior. Some are benign and of local significance, whereas others are highly malignant and metastasize to regional lymph nodes and lungs. Treatment is usually surgical removal as these neoplasms are not radiosensitive. In the benign variety the prognosis is good, whereas in the malignant variety the prognosis is poor.

Ameloblastoma is one of the special epithelial neoplasms arising in the oral region (Fig. 78). Ameloblastoma arises from epithelial elements of the enamel organ and because of this origin it is sometimes designated a developmental neoplasm. In most instances, it develops within the jaw, most often in the third molar region of the mandible of patients about 30 years of age. It has been reported as early as three years of age and as late as 70 years, but the average age of occurrence is 30 years.

Ameloblastoma, often erroneously termed adamantinoma, grows

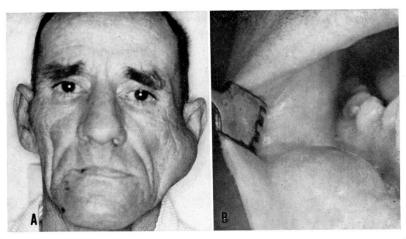

Figure 77. *Tumors.* A, Swelling of mid-lateral face is typical of parotid gland tumor. B, Dome-like swelling of vestibular mucosa is produced by a tumor of accessory salivary glands.

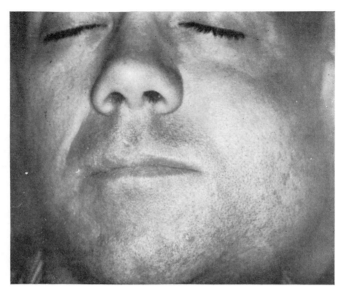

Figure 78. *Ameloblastoma.* Smooth swelling associated with the angle of the jaw is typical of ameloblastoma.

in proliferating buds resembling the enamel organ or dental lamina so that it has a tendency to extend through the marrow spaces. It also has a strong tendency to become cystic causing it to be expansile. With the development of a cystic pattern, it produces local swelling and deformity of the face, which in advanced cases may be extensive. Although the neoplasm has some tendency to invade locally, it remains well differentiated and does not metastasize. Some reports of metastasis appear in the literature, but most of these are to the lung in patients who have undergone repeated incomplete surgical removal. They probably represent spread by aspiration rather than true metastasis.

Ameloblastoma is treated by surgery as the neoplasm is not radiosensitive. Its pattern of growth necessitates wide surgical excision and sometimes resection of the jaw. Because of its tendency to extend through the marrow spaces and sometimes its incomplete removal, the neoplasm frequently recurs and may have to be removed several times. In spite of repeated recurrences, the neoplasm rarely kills the patient even when there is evidence that it has spread to the lungs.

Neoplasms of Mesenchymal Origin

The mesenchymal neoplasms, with the exception of odontomas, are rare in the oral region and odontomas are not too common.

Benign mesenchymal tumors occur more frequently than the malignant ones. This finding is fortunate, because sarcomas of the head and neck region have a very poor prognosis, in fact, they are rarely cured. Only the most commonly occurring mesenchymal neoplasms are discussed briefly in this book.

Lipoma is a tumor composed of adipose tissue and occurs in all parts of the body where there is fat (Fig. 79). It is, therefore, a tumor which occurs in many anatomic locations. In the oral region it occurs in the buccal fat pads of the cheek and the floor of the mouth as an indistinct, smooth, soft swelling. When the tumor is just beneath the mucosa in the floor of the mouth, the yellow color of the fat may show through the thin mucosa. Lipomas grow slowly, remain benign, and are easily treated surgically.

Fibromas are composed of fibrous connective tissue and may occur in the lips, tongue, palate, gingiva, and jaws (Fig. 80). They are usually slow-growing nodular lesions which become pedunculated when near the surface. The overlying mucosa is more pale than normal tissue, and the lesion is more firm than normal tissue. Fibromas are easily cured by complete local excision.

Tumors arising from *nervous* tissue are rarely pure tumors, but are composed of nerve tissue and fibrous tissue. Either tissue may predominate and any element of the nerve may be present. When

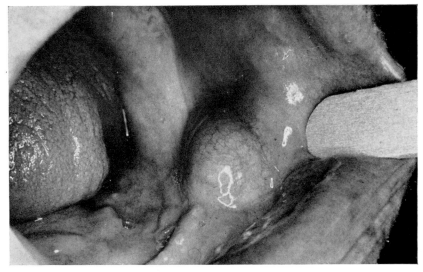

Figure 79. *Lipoma*. Smooth nodular mass in the buccal mucosa is yellowish in color. The tortuous capillaries are evident on the surface because the mucosa is stretched. The mass is poorly circumscribed and easily compressible on palpation.

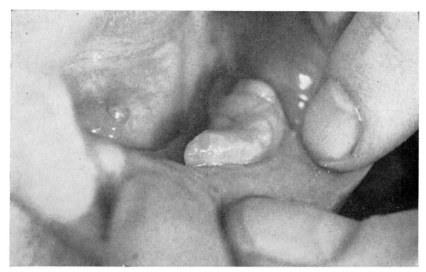

Figure 80. *Fibroma.* The crescentric lesion extending from the lower alveolar ridge is slightly lighter than the normal mucosa. It is firm in consistency and solidly fixed to the mandible.

the nerve elements grow as nerve fibers in fibrous tissue, they are called cirsoid *neurofibromas,* the most common variety seen in the oral region. Neurofibromas occur in the lips, buccal mucosa, tongue, and occasionally in the jaw. They produce a nodular swelling, which may exhibit pain because the nerve fibers are functional. Other tumors of nervous tissue origin may arise from the elements of the nerve sheath which become intermingled with the fibrous tissue. Such tumors are called neurilemmomas or Schwannomas. They are less common than the cirsoid variety and are not painful, as the nerve elements are sheath cells rather than neurons. Both types of tumors grow slowly and produce limited symptoms other than local deformity. One variety of neurofibroma occurs as a developmental tumor in the tongue of infants and is designated a congenital neurofibroma. It causes marked enlargement of the tongue and may extend into the neck. All types of fibroma are treated by surgery and the results are excellent, except in congenital neurofibroma which holds a poor prognosis when the whole tongue is involved or when the neoplasm extends into the neck.

Hemangioma and *lymphangioma* (angiomas) occur in the oral cavity; the former are by far the more frequent. Angiomas occur in the lips, buccal mucosa, tongue, and occasionally in the substance of the jaw (Fig. 81A, B, C). The tumors are composed of vascular structures varying in size from a capillary to very large endothelial-

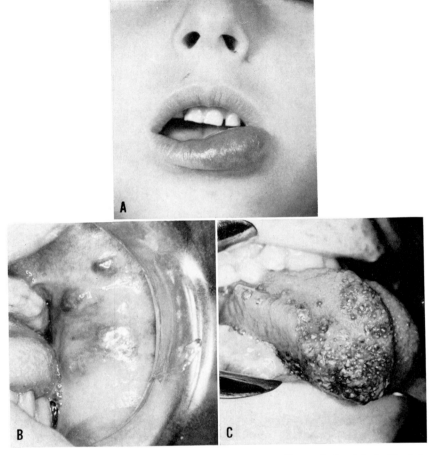

Figure 81. *Hemangioma.* A, The smooth dark swelling of the left half of the lower lip is a hemangioma of the type often present in children. B, Numerous dark nodules of buccal mucosa are due to cavernous hemangioma. C, Numerous small nodules on dorsum and lateral tongue present one pattern of hemangioma of the tongue.

lined spaces. The appearance of the lesion is dependent upon the size of the vascular spaces. Those composed of numerous capillaries are slightly elevated, bright-red lesions of small size, usually not more than a centimeter in diameter. Those composed of very large vascular spaces are elevated, nodular, bluish masses, which may be from a centimeter to several inches in area. The large tumors are soft, and pulsations may be felt on palpation if they are closely associated with an artery.

Angiomas of the tongue are sometimes congenital and produce marked macroglossia. The congenital angiomas of the tongue may extend into the neck and involve it extensively. Angiomas of varying color and size may involve the skin of the face and lip and extend through the full thickness of the lips and cheeks. On the skin they are called "birthmarks" or "port wine stains." Small angiomas may be surgically excised with a cure, but removal of large ones is difficult and may necessitate skin grafts to repair the defect. Congenital angiomas of the tongue and floor of the mouth have a poor prognosis because of the extensive involvement and the difficulty of removal. Large tumors are sometimes reduced in size by the use of sclerosing solutions before surgery is attempted. The injection of sclerosing solutions causes thrombosis and obliteration of the vascular spaces by scarring. After the spaces are obliterated the residual scarred tumor is excised.

Odontomas are tumors arising from tooth-forming elements, either of mesenchymal or epithelial and mesenchymal elements. Those arising from only the epithelial elements have already been discussed under ameloblastomas. Odontogenic neoplasms of mesenchymal origin are the *odontogenic myxomas* which arise from the dental papilla and the *odontogenic fibromas* which arise from the dental sac. The odontogenic myxoma and odontogenic fibroma are rare benign tumors arising in the portion of the jaw where a tooth is missing. They grow slowly and expand the jaw but usually present no other symptoms. The tumors are treated successfully by surgical removal.

The majority of the odontogenic tumors are derived from both epithelial and mesenchymal elements with varying proportions of both tissues being represented in different tumors. In some odontogenic tumors the epithelial elements predominate, whereas in others the epithelium is very sparse. Some of these tumors form calcified enamel and dentin and are called hard or calcified mixed odontogenic tumors. In contrast to those which are not differentiated to such a level that they can produce calcifiable enamel or dentin are the soft or noncalcified mixed odontogenic tumors. Some of the calcified tumors are composed almost entirely of enamel and dentin in varied proportions and arrangement. Some investigators believe that this is a maturing process and that eventually all of the noncalcified tumors will reach this state. Both the soft and calcified mixed odontogenic tumors are benign, slow-growing, and can be successfully treated surgically.

Odontogenic tumors composed almost entirely of calcified tissue are called *composite odontomas*. When the tumor tissue exhibits only histodifferentiation and the enamel and dentin do not simulate

10

the arrangement of a tooth, it is called a *complex composite odontoma*. When the tumor exhibits both histo- and morphodifferentiation and the enamel and dentin have the arrangement of miniature teeth, the tumor is designated a *compound composite odontoma* (Fig. 82). Both of these types of odontoma are benign, slow-growing tumors which can be treated successfully surgically.

Malignant mesenchymal neoplasms of all types may involve the jaw, but the incidence is very low for all types. The fibrosarcoma and osteogenic sarcomas are the most frequent primary malignant mesenchymal neoplasms of the oral region, while the neoplasms of lymphoid tissue origin are the most common variety which are

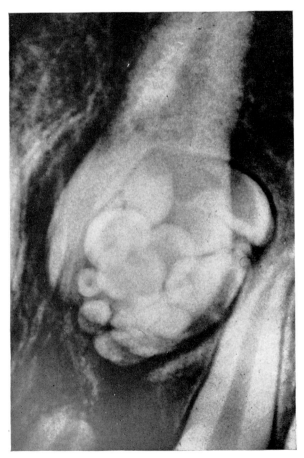

Figure 82. *Compound composite odontoma.* Several small calcified structures representative of miniature teeth are contained in a radiolucent area surrounded by a connective tissue membrane.

primary in the neck. All of the malignant mesenchymal neoplasms in the head and neck region have a grave prognosis because they present difficult treatment problems in that they are not radiosensitive and are difficult to remove completely by surgery. The malignant mesenchymal tumors have a decided tendency to metastasize by the hematogenous route, and, therefore, the metastatic lesions are more remote and extensive.

Metastatic neoplasms of both epithelial and mesenchymal origin may involve the oral region, especially the jaws. The most common metastatic neoplasm found in the jaws is carcinoma of the breast, which has a marked tendency to metastasize to bone, and often the jaw is the site of metastasis. Carcinoma of the thyroid and prostate likewise metastasize to bone and may occur in the jaw. Metastatic tumors of the jaw have a poor prognosis since the primary neoplasm is elsewhere, and even though the lesion of the jaw is eliminated, the patient is not free of the disease and may ultimately be killed by the primary neoplasm.

The possibility of the presence of neoplasm should always be kept in mind and the patient directed for treatment. Early recognition and treatment may save a life.

BIBLIOGRAPHY

Blum, H. F.: Sunlight as a causal factor in cancer of the skin of man. J. Nat. Cancer Inst., 9:247, 1948.

Dorn, H. F., and Cutler, S. J.: Morbidity from cancer in the United States. Public Health Monograph No. 29, U.S. Public Health Service, pt. 2, 1955.

Fine, G., Marshall, R. B., and Horn, R. C.: Tumors of minor salivary glands. Cancer, 13:653, 1963.

Foote, F. W., and Frazell, E. H.: Tumors of major salivary glands. Cancer, 6:1065, 1953.

Hopps, H. .C.: Principles of Pathology. New York, Appleton-Century-Crofts, Inc., 1959.

Kerr, D. A.: Keratotic lesions of the oral cavity. J. Dent. Med., 13:92, 1958.

Potdar, G. G., and Paymaster, J. C.: Tumors of minor salivary glands. Oral Surg., 28:310, 1969.

Smith, J. F.: Salivary gland lesions—variations and predictability. Oral Surg., 27:499, 1969.

Spouge, J. D.: Odontogenic tumors. Oral Surg., 24:392, 1967.

Chapter 6
RETROGRESSIVE CHANGES AND METABOLIC DISTURBANCES

TYPES OF RETROGRESSIVE CHANGES

Retrogressive changes involve atrophy, degenerations, infiltrations, concretions, deposits, and "degenerative" changes that impair tissue function. These changes, in contrast to progressive changes, are not altruistic. Retrogressive changes reflect the response of cells to an adverse environment which causes cellular injury. The most complete form of retrogressive change is death, both local cell death and somatic death of the whole organism.

Retrogressive changes may also be considered as "wear-and-tear" changes. Retrograde changes result in a decrease in the functional capacity of cells and a reduction in the efficiency of organs, parts, or the entire organism. In this respect these changes are analogous to the wearing-out of the parts of a machine. The same is true of the human organism, wherein wear and tear of a part of the body results in a decrease in functional efficiency of cells and disease of that part occurs. When the loss of function is severe enough, the entire organism may be affected to such a degree that continued life is impossible and death results. Death also may be due to a combination of retrogressive changes in several parts of the organism.

Some retrogressive changes start at birth, or before, and progress throughout the lifetime of the individual. The progressive "downward" changes occurring throughout life are also the changes of aging and are significant forms of disease. They may be intensified in extent and rate of change by factors in the environment, i.e., by extrinsic factors responsible for disease. They may also be of increased importance to the organism where there are hereditary or developmental alterations upon which the retrogressive changes are superimposed.

Attrition is a constant form of retrogressive change seen in teeth. Attrition is the wearing-away of teeth as the result of mastication

(Fig. 83). It occurs on the occlusal, incisal, and interproximal surfaces. Attrition increases with age and may be influenced by the abrasive quality of the diet and by habits of mastication. The first sign of attrition is the development of small flat smooth surfaces where the teeth rub together. In extreme wear the full thickness of the enamel may be worn away with the exposure of dentin which has a marked tendency to absorb stain from food or tobacco. This stains the dentin light to dark brown. In extreme cases the crown of the tooth may be almost completely worn away. With excessive wear the teeth do not function efficiently in the mastication of food.

Abrasion (Fig. 84) refers to the act of abrading—the wear produced by some abnormal mechanical processes. The location and pattern of wear are dependent upon the cause. Notches are seen in the incisal edge of incisors as the result of opening bobby pins, biting thread, and holding tacks or other objects between the teeth. It is also produced in patients who have the habit of grinding their teeth (bruxism). Habits such as chewing tobacco or betel nuts result in

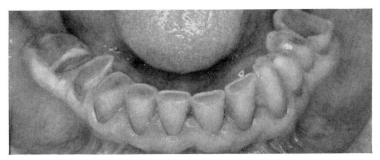

Figure 83. *Attrition.* Excessive occlusal and incisal wear associated with chewing tobacco.

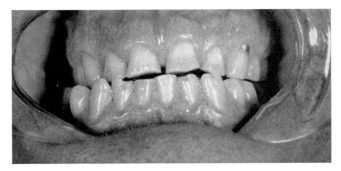

Figure 84. *Occupational abrasion.* Excessive incisal wear associated with glassblowing.

intense wear in selected areas. Interproximal abrasion may be produced by the incorrect use of toothpicks and dental floss. The wear produced by floss is usually a narrow groove on the mesial and distal surfaces just above the gum margin. When produced by toothpicks, the wear is a saucer-shaped lesion on the interproximal surface of two adjacent teeth. Abrasion may be produced by the improper brushing of teeth using a hard brush and an abrasive dentifrice (Fig. 85). This results when the brushing stroke is horizontal and the abrasion occurs as a notch just above the gingival margin of the buccal and labial surfaces. The process is usually more severe on one side than on the other depending upon whether the individual is right- or left-handed. The most severe abrasion appears on the side opposite to the hand holding the brush. In very severe cases the notching may extend one-third to one-half of the thickness of the tooth and so weaken the tooth that it may break off at the gingival margin.

Erosion is a process characterized by the loss of tooth substance through demineralization which occurs on the labial surface of maxillary incisors and the cervical region of bicuspids and molars without apparent cause (idiopathic erosion). It is also produced in other locations from habitually sucking on citrus fruits, ingestion of highly acid medicaments, habitual regurgitation of stomach contents, or inhalation of acid fumes.

The lesions in idiopathic erosion are trench-like lesions with smooth glistening bases appearing to have been produced by something flowing over the tooth surface. In cases produced by the presence of acid, the changes are loss of enamel and dentin from the surfaces contacted by the acid. The surface is hard and glistening in contrast to caries in which it is soft and discolored (Fig. 86).

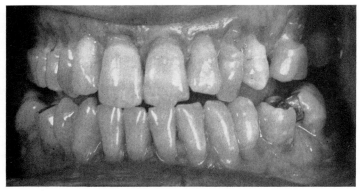

Figure 85. *Abrasion.* Deep cervical notches due to vigorous brushing with a horizontal stroke.

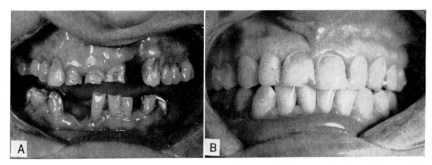

Figure 86. *Erosion.* A, Extensive loss of enamel due to habitually sucking
    lemons. B, Idiopathic erosion showing cupping at the cervical area
    and ditching of the labial incisal area.

Resorption of teeth is a retrogressive change which may occur
from within (internal resorption) or it may start on the root surface
(external resorption). Resorption of teeth is associated with inflammation, excessive function, and the presence of tumors near the
roots of the teeth. The entire root surface may be resorbed and the
tooth lost. Internal resorption of the crown produces a pink spot
which appears to be in the enamel but is due to the resorption of
the underlying dentin (Fig. 87A, B, D). The enamel may also be
resorbed and the pulp exposed necessitating extraction of the tooth
or endodontic therapy.

Atrophy

Atrophy is a retrogressive change characterized by a reduction in
the size of cells or a decrease in the total number of cells present in
mature tissue or a fully formed organ (Fig. 49). Atrophy may be
due to disuse of a part, starvation, pressure, toxins, infections, or
irradiation. The most striking example of disuse atrophy is that
associated with the paralysis of muscles from poliomyelitis. Similarly
diminished activity or function of a tissue is followed by atrophy.
Continued pressure upon a tissue produces atrophy either by affecting the cells directly or by interfering with the blood supply of the
tissue. Toxins and infections may produce atrophy of parenchymatous tissue, viz., atrophy of submaxillary gland associated with an
infected salivary calculus in the gland duct. Atrophy of the skin
and glandular tissue may be present in association with x-ray irradiation. In these instances parenchymatous or glandular tissue is
usually replaced by fibrous connective tissue.

Atrophy frequently accompanies age, decreased functional demand, and reduced nutrition. Atrophy of the vermilion border of
the lip occurs in older individuals due in part to aging and in part

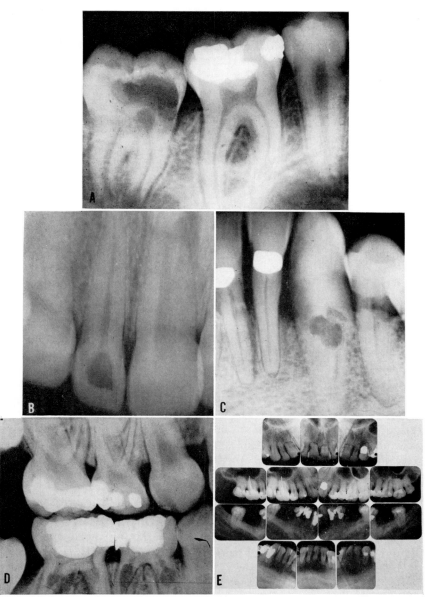

Figure 87. *Internal and external resorption.* A, Internal resorption in the crown of a second molar. B, Marked enlargement of the coronal pulp of a maxillary lateral incisor. Because the vascular pulp shows through the thinned enamel as a pink spot, these teeth are called pink teeth. C, Irregular resorption in mid-root of a mandibular cuspid. In some cases this resorption is initiated externally and in others internally. D, Internal resorption of deciduous molars following pulpotomy. E, Root resorption especially marked in the maxillary incisors.

to exposure of the lip to sunlight. In this instance the surface epithelium is atrophic and becomes thin and shiny. The lip becomes opaque owing to alteration in keratin metabolism which is also a retrogressive change in squamous epithelium. This condition is called solar or senile cheilitis. Atrophy may occur with age in the tongue and the cheeks. The connective tissue and muscle are reduced in amount and partially replaced by fat. Such a replacement is called fatty atrophy. This results in decrease in size and loss of tissue tone. Atrophy also occurs in the salivary glands with age. In this instance also the gland cells are replaced by fat which results in diminished function. The reduced output of saliva produces dryness of the mouth (xerostomia). Xerostomia is not uncommon in elderly patients and is a source of annoyance since it is uncomfortable and makes eating and speaking difficult. Nutritional atrophy is discussed in Chapter 5.

Degenerations

Degeneration refers to those alterations of cells due to the direct action of injurious agents and to secondary changes resulting from an altered intracellular metabolism caused by the injury. Degeneration of many body cells is a daily occurrence due to the "wear and tear" of injury, functional demand, and, to some extent, aging. Degenerative changes may be reversed if alteration of the cells has not progressed too far, otherwise death of the cells occurs. Degenerations are present in a variety of conditions and usually produce some reduction in efficiency. Minimal degenerative changes in one part of the body may be of little significance to the organism as far as survival is concerned, but the summation of all the degenerative changes in all of the organs and parts of the body may make survival impossible.

Disturbances in metabolism of epithelial tissues may be associated with areas of mechanical, thermal, or chemical irritation resulting in increased keratinization of the epithelium. These retrogressive changes may be associated with cheek-chewing, smoking, the use of irritating mouthwashes, and dentifrices. Specific processes of this nature are discussed in Chapter 12 on stomatitis, page 250.

DEGENERATION INVOLVING PROTEINS. Certain diseases disturb intracellular protein metabolism which result in cellular degenerations. The various types of protein degenerations include cloudy swelling, hydropic degeneration, hyaline degeneration, amyloidosis, and mucoprotein accumulations. *Cloudy swelling* represents subtle cytoplasmic protein changes resulting in granularity and cloudiness of the cytoplasm of the cells. Such changes are most evident in the parenchymal cells, especially of the kidney, heart, and liver, in response to febrile illness, malnutrition, and poisoning. The cause of degeneration is the result of some toxic substance in the environment of the cell which, due to protein alteration, causes the cell to acquire more fluid. The presence of toxins produced by microorganisms, the catabolic products associated with fever, or some other dilute toxin produces this mild form of degeneration which may be reversible.

Hydropic degeneration is a progressive state of cloudy swelling, and it is questionable as to whether or not it is reversible. When intense it produces necrosis. The degeneration is characterized by the formation of cytoplasmic vacuoles apparently due to the inhibition of water into the cell as the result of injury. This type of degeneration is present in liver cells following exposure to certain anesthetics and chemical solvents, such as carbon tetrachloride.

Hyaline degeneration refers to retrogressive changes that result in the cytoplasm taking on a homogeneous translucent, glassy appearance. The term "hyaline" is a descriptive term and refers to the physical appearance of the altered cytoplasm. Hyaline degeneration is a defect of the metabolism of cytoplasmic proteins in either epithelium or connective tissue. Hyalinization of the walls of blood vessels is characteristic of certain types of arteriosclerosis and of the vessels of atrophic ovaries and uteri following menopause. The term *hyaline* is sometimes used to describe the appearance of the cornified layer of squamous epithelial cells, dense old scar tissue, and the connective tissue of old mature dental pulps. While the appearances of such tissue probably do not represent a true degeneration but an effect of aging or involutionary changes, they are often included in hyaline degeneration because they simulate the histologic and staining features of hyaline degeneration.

Amyloidosis is the deposition of hyalin-like material between parenchymal cells and in connective tissue. There are several forms of amyloidosis but they are usually grouped, for convenience and pathogenesis, into primary and secondary forms. Secondary amyloidosis is the most common form and is associated most often with chronic infections, especially of bone, with the deposition of amyloid in kidneys, spleen, and liver. Primary amyloidosis apparently occurs in the absence of predisposing factors and is found most often in the muscles of the tongue and heart.

Combinations of protein and carbohydrate (mucoproteins, mucopolysaccharides) make up a group of chemical substances elaborated by epithelial and connective tissue cells. One such substance is *mucin* which is secreted by epithelial cells lining mucosal surfaces; a similar material, *mucoid,* may be elaborated by mesenchymal elements. Mucinous degeneration is often used to designate the presence of an excess of mucin. Although such an excess is not considered a true degeneration, it is often found interstitially with cellular degeneration. The production of excessive amounts of mucin is characteristic of catarrhal inflammation associated with the common cold. The retention of mucus because of ductal obstruction leads to the formation of mucoceles, viz., retention cysts of accessory salivary glands (Fig. 88). Myxomas, tumors arising from myxomatous connective tissue, elaborate abundant mucoid. Abnormal accumulations of mucopolysaccharides occur in the *"collagen diseases,"* viz., rheumatic fever, rheumatoid arthritis.

The ground substance of connective tissue is rich in mucopolysaccharides (hyaluronic acid, chondroitin-sulfuric acid) and therefore is important in the tissue integrity of the periodontal membrane. Certain bacteria present in the mouth are capable of producing *hyaluronidase,* an enzyme capable of hydrolizing mucopolysaccharides. The elaboration of such an enzyme (hyaluronidase) in the gingival crevice is an important factor in the loss of the integrity of the principal fibers of the periodontal membrane, the spread of inflammation, and the production of periodontal pockets. (See Periodontitis, Chapter 11, p. 237.)

DEGENERATIONS INVOLVING LIPIDS. Disease processes may alter the quantity and distribution of the lipids found in tissue cells. Normally lipid is present in the cells in two forms. Visible stainable fat is present in special types of cells called fat cells. These cells store lipid material in a labile form which can be available for utilization on need. Aggregates of fat cells are distributed throughout the body as adipose tissue. The second type of lipid is a part of the cytoplasm of the cell. It is an intimate part of the protoplasm and is invisible in the cell. Two alterations may occur in the metabolism of lipid, fatty degeneration and degenerative fatty infiltration.

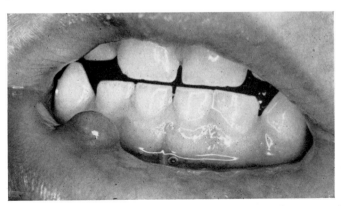

Figure 88. Mucocele due to the retention of mucin in the tissue following injury to the lip.

Fatty degeneration is the appearance of stainable lipid in cells or organs in which lipid normally cannot be demonstrated. The lipid occurs in the cell as the result of severe parenchymatous degeneration with separation of the lipid from the cytoplasm to appear in droplets of varying size within the cells. Such change is evidence of injury produced by exotoxins of microorganisms, by poisons, and in severe anoxia. The heart and kidneys are most often and severely affected.

Degenerative fatty infiltration is produced by mild cellular degeneration which causes liver cells to accumulate lipid transported from some other area of the body. Owing to minor cell injury, parenchymal cells may accumluate large quantities of lipid that they are unable to metabolize. The accumulation of lipid in tissue produces an increase in size of the organ or tissue and may replace parenchyma contributing to the reduced function produced by the degeneration. Fatty infiltration and fatty degeneration are sometimes referred to as fatty metamorphosis. Lipid may also accumulate in organs and tissues as fat cells replacing normal parenchyma and is designated fatty atrophy.

Infiltrations

The term *infiltration* refers to the accumulation of metabolites within healthy cells due to metabolic derangements of systemic origin. Infiltrations involve lipids and carbohydrates. Infiltration differs from degeneration in the factors which lead up to these regressive changes. The accumulation of metabolites in degeneration follows injury, whereas in infiltration the accumulation of metabolites in healthy cells produces the injury.

Lipids. *Fatty atrophy* is the replacement of tissue by fat, especially parenchymal tissue that has undergone marked atrophy. Fatty atrophy occurs in salivary glands, thymus, pancreas, and heart. Aging and obesity are important predisposing factors in fatty atrophy of the heart. While the adult fat cells do not reproduce themselves to fill in spaces caused by tissue atrophy, existing mesenchymal tissue accumulates lipids to form adult fat cells. Thus, in obesity, there is an increase in lipids and an increased number of adult fat cells present which store the lipids provided by an excess of food intake over body requirements. The infiltration and accumulation of labile fat (extracellular fat) in healthy parenchymal cells are, for practical purposes, limited to the liver. This condition is designated *fatty infiltration* and may occur in chronic alcoholism, malnutrition, and wasting diseases. The most common cause of fatty change in the liver is a dietary deficiency of lipotropics, viz., choline, lecithin, and riboflavin.

CARBOHYDRATES. The abnormal accumulation of glycogen in the cells of the body reflects hyperglycemia with the exception of one rather uncommon disease involving glycogen storage. The most severe infiltration of glycogen is found in diabetes mellitus. Diabetes mellitus is a disturbance in the utilization of carbohydrate and is evidenced by an increase in sugar in urine and blood. The etiology is unknown, although heredity and obesity appear to be important factors. This disease has a high incidence, occurs more frequently in women than in men, and develops most often in the fifth and sixth decades of life. Diabetes is one of the ten major causes of death; it has been estimated that there are approximately one million persons in the United States with this disease. The disordered carbohydrate metabolism basically results from a deficiency in insulin or from the action of insulin. Well-established diabetes mellitus is characterized by excessive appetite, excessive thirst, general weakness, and polyuria. In advanced cases degenerative changes, such as cataracts, generalized arteriosclerosis, infections, and gangrene involving the feet and toes, occur. Diabetic patients may develop multiple periodontal abscesses.

Disturbances in glycogen storage (Von Gierke's disease) is an inborn defect in glycogen metabolism, especially of infants, with large quantities retained in liver, kidney, and heart.

URIC ACID. Certain individuals have a limited altered metabolism of uric acid obtained from animal nucleoproteins. The uric acid is deposited in the kidneys and in joint capsules. The deposition in joint capsules and ligaments provides a swollen tender or painful joint due to the accumulation of uric acid crystals in the tissue. The process is designated as gout. Crystals of uric acid may also be deposited in the subcutaneous tissues and produce nodular swellings (tophi).

Necrosis

Necrosis is local cell death due to disease or injury. Cell death is a dynamic process, not an instantaneous occurrence, and involves both nuclear and cytoplasmic changes. Although basic morphologic alterations occur in the death of all cells, specific alterations of cellular structure may be recognized if specific cells are affected and if certain injurious agents are responsible for cellular death. Thus, the following specific types of necrosis may be found: coagulation, liquefaction, caseation, and gangrenous necrosis.

Coagulation necrosis refers to the local death of cells in which the protein elements of the cytoplasm become fixed and opaque by coagulation. An intercellular form of this type of necrosis (Fig. 89A, B) is the pseudomembrane of Vincent's infection (acute necrotizing

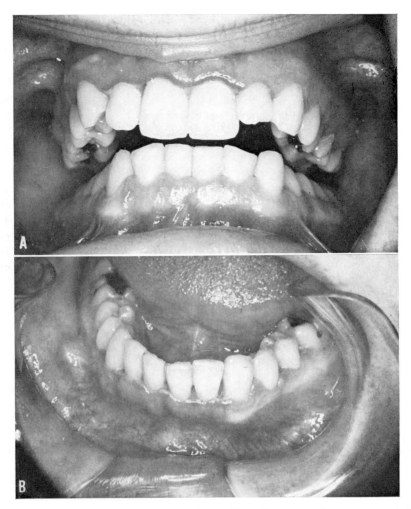

Figure 89. A, *Necrosis* of interdental papillae of incisors due to necrotizing ulcerative gingivitis. The pseudomembrane of the process is well shown in the right maxillary lateral incisor area. B, Residual interproximal defect in chronic necrotizing ulcerative gingivitis.

gingivitis). *Liquefaction* necrosis is a type of necrosis in which there is a fairly rapid nonbacterial, enzymatic dissolution and destruction of whole cells. This cellular alteration results in the production of fluid. An example of this type of necrosis is seen in the liquefaction of cells and the formation of pus in a periodontal abscess. *Caseation* necrosis refers to the conversion of dead cells into a soft, friable, cottage-cheese-like mass. It is seen most commonly in association with tuberculosis. *Gangrenous* necrosis has all the basic features of simple necrosis plus those changes associated with the invasion of saprophytes. Several forms of gangrene may be encountered: dry, moist, and gas gangrene.

Dry gangrene is the result of altered and reduced circulation in a part with poor or no collateral circulation. It is produced in the extremities by freezing, diabetes, and arteriosclerosis. It may occur in the dental pulp when a severe blow disrupts the vessels at the apex of the tooth.

Moist gangrene is produced by reduced and altered circulation of parts which have a good collateral circulation so that fluid is supplied to the necrotic tissue. This form of necrosis is seen in the lung and the gut and occurs in the pulp with carious exposure. Gas gangrene is most often seen in the extremities associated with serious wounds contaminated with B. welchii.

Necrosis of the dental pulp occurs as the result of carious exposure or altered pulpal circulation due to trauma. Necrosis of the dental pulp is discussed in Chapter 9, page 185.

METABOLIC DISTURBANCES

Mineral Metabolism

Mineral infiltration and concretions are primarily concerned with the metabolism and deposition of calcium salts. Pathologic calcification is the presence of abnormal calcific deposits within the soft tissues of the body. The deposition of calcium salts in soft tissues as a result of an increased amount of calcium in the blood is termed *metastatic calcification*. Metastatic calcification may occur with hypervitaminosis D related to the excessive intake of irradiated milk or vitamin D concentrates. Pathologic calcifications secondary to injured degenerating or dead tissue is termed *dystrophic calcification*. The formation of concretions of solid materials in hollow spaces, tubes, or body crevices is termed *lithiasis*. The deposition of calcium in organic matrix gives rise to hard stony calculi. Such calcareous deposits occur primarily in the biliary ducts, collecting system of the kidneys, and in the ducts of the salivary glands. The formation of salivary calculi (sialoliths) in the ducts of salivary glands is referred to as sialolithiasis. The obstruction of salivary gland ducts by salivary calculi causes dilatation of the duct and chronic inflammation of the entire gland. The obstruction of the duct and the accumulation of saliva give rise to a retention cyst. Such a cyst in the floor of the mouth is often termed a ranula (Fig. 90). The formation of gallstones and kidney stones are other examples of the process of lithiasis.

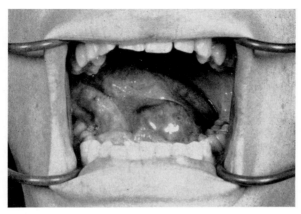

Figure 90. Mucous retention cyst (ranula) of sublingual gland due to an obstruction produced by a sialolith.

With advancing age calcium salts are deposited in the dentinal tubules making the dentin more dense. The process of deposition of calcium salts into a noncalcified tissue, such as a dentinal tubule or blood vessel, is called sclerosis and the involved structure is said to be sclerotic. Sclerosis of dentin is seen in almost all teeth with advancing age and produces a change in the color of teeth. The teeth become more yellow and less translucent. The darkening of teeth with age is often of concern to the patient but cannot be prevented or decreased by any form of treatment.

All teeth undergo regressive changes with age in that calcium salts are deposited in both the radicular and coronal areas of the pulp. In the crown these deposits are spherical in form and are called denticles or *pulp stones* (Fig. 91). In the radicular area the calcium is deposited in a diffuse pattern (Fig. 92). The spherical masses in the crown can be visualized by x-ray films, but unless extensive the radicular calcification is not readily demonstrated. Accompanying the pulpal calcification there is also a progressive fibrosis or aging of the pulp. These changes reduce the vitality of the pulp and do not permit the old pulp to repair with the same facility as the young pulp. Pulp stones rarely produce pain and are of little significance unless root canal procedures are indicated. The presence of pulp stones may preclude endodontic procedures.

The formation of calcareous deposits on the teeth is discussed in Chapter 10 on stain and accretions, page 202.

Iron is an important element in the biosynthesis of hemoglobin and a deficiency or an excess of this element may give rise to disease states. A deficiency of iron may occur from an inadequate dietary

11

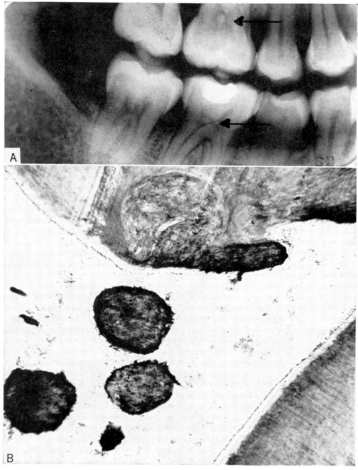

Figure 91. *Denticles (pulp stones)*. A, Radiograph of pulp stones in pulp chamber of maxillary first molar. B, Spherical masses in coronal pulp.

intake associated with bizarre diets; inadequate absorption encountered in advanced age and intestinal disease; and excessive losses of iron as the result of chronic blood loss, viz., chronic hemorrhage associated with carcinoma of the gastrointestinal tract, menstruation, and pregnancy. Deficiencies of iron prevent adequate formation of hemoglobin and lead to iron deficiency anemias. An excess of iron resulting in iron accumulation in the body may occur from excessive destruction of red blood cells. Such a condition occurs in the hemolytic anemias.

Iodine is necessary for the normal function of the thyroid gland.

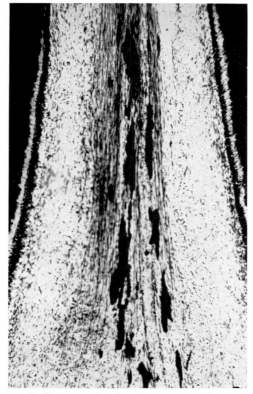

Figure 92. Linear calcification of radicular portion of pulp. Calcium salts deposited in linear masses along path of vessels.

A dietary deficiency of this element occurs in areas where vegetables are grown in soil containing little or no iodine. A deficiency of iodine results in endemic goiter. The addition of iodine to table salt has done much to eliminate this disease.

Disturbances of *fluorine* metabolism of the teeth are discussed in Chapter 8 on dental caries. Fluorine is a very toxic substance and, when ingested, is stored in calcified tissues. It is eliminated slowly by the kidneys. Excessive amounts of fluorine produce skeletal and renal disease and mottled enamel.

ARTERIOSCLEROSIS.   While the term arteriosclerosis actually means hardening of the arteries, it includes several variants which have in common the thickening and loss of elasticity of arterial walls; however, the variants differ in etiology and pathogenesis. The three variants of arteriosclerosis include: (1) *atherosclerosis,* characterized by the deposition of lipids in the subendothelial connective tissue of the intima of arterial walls; (2) *medial calcific sclerosis,* characterized by calcification of the media of muscular arteries; and (3) *hyperplastic arteriolosclerosis,* characterized by hyperplastic thickening of the walls of small arteries and arterioles.

The most important form of arteriosclerosis is atherosclerosis and is the most common form of primary vascular disease. The high incidence of atherosclerosis with frequent involvement of the blood supply to the heart, kidneys, and brain accounts in part for the dominant position of cardiovascular disease as the cause of death in this country. Atherosclerosis causes deformity, narrowing of the lumen, and occlusion of arteries and predisposes to ischemia, atrophy, and infarction of dependent structures supplied by the involved vessels. Involvement of such dependent structures as the brain, especially areas of cerebral function involving judgment, memory, and personality, are particularly vulnerable. In addition to ischemia resulting from the narrowing of vascular lumens, an infarction in the brain may occur as a result of vascular occlusion due to thrombosis superimposed upon atheromatous changes. Cerebral hemorrhage is a serious consequence of atherosclerosis. Hemorrhage and thrombosis are often associated with atherosclerosis and for this reason the presence of atherosclerosis of the coronary vessels of the heart is an important predisposing cause of cardiac infarcts. There is some evidence to indicate that low fat diets, particularly those low in cholesterol, may be helpful in the prevention and treatment of the early stages of atherosclerosis and thus prevent the effects of atherosclerosis, viz., death due to sequelae of coronary occlusion.

Pigment Metabolism

The term *pigment* refers to a wide variety of chemical deposits formed *within* the body due to abnormal or normal functional activity (endogenous pigments), or their accumulation from *outside* the body due to inhalation or absorption (exogenous pigments). Pigments in general give rise to gross or microscopic discoloration of the tissues involved.

Exogenous pigments include coal dust, metallic silver, and iron dust. The accumulations of coal or iron dusts in the lungs and draining lymphatic tissues in miners are occupational hazards. The deposition of silver may occur from prolonged use of medicaments containing silver salts. Silver pigmentation (argyria) gives the skin and mucous membranes a gray-blue discoloration (Fig. 93). Localized argyrosis occurs in the gingiva usually from the inadvertent deposition of silver amalgam fragments into alveolar sockets during extraction of teeth. Bismuth pigmentation also occurs rarely (Fig. 94).

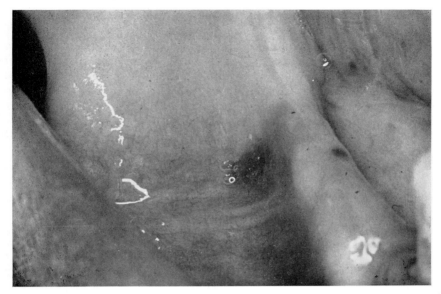

Figure 93. *Argyrosis*. Bluish spots in the buccal mucosa and the alveolar ridge are associated with the implantation of particles of amalgam in the tissue.

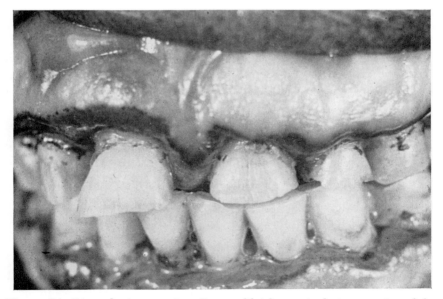

Figure 94. *Bismuth pigmentation*. Intense bluish marginal pigmentation of the gingiva due to bismuth administration as a part of antiluetic therapy. Heavy calculus deposits are evident and contribute to the marginal irritation and deposition of bismuth salts.

Endogenous pigments are almost entirely derived from the breakdown of hemoglobin. Melanin is an important pigment which is not derived from hemoglobin. In conditions where there is an increased destruction of red cells as in the hemolytic anemias, iron pigment may accumulate in certain tissues of the body, especially those of the reticuloendothelial system and in macrophages of the skin and mucous membranes. Localized iron pigmentation occurs in focal areas of hemorrhage. One pigment not derived from hemoglobin, porphyrin, may occur in excess (rare) and give rise to red deposits in the teeth and other tissues.

Pigments related to bile, especially bilirubin, are normally excreted in the bile. Bilirubinogenous pigments, when present in excess in the blood plasma, cause *jaundice* (icterus). Icterus may occur as the result of excess hemolysis of red blood cells, liver disease, and obstruction of the bile ducts. Melanin is an endogenous pigment normally present in the choroid coat of the eye, oral mucous membrane, and skin. It is produced by specialized cells in the basal layer of the epidermis and imparts color to the skin. The amount of melanin is increased by exposure to sunlight and prevents penetration of ultraviolet light. Tanning is a function of increased melanin production due to exposure especially to actinic irradiation. Increased pigmentation of skin and oral mucosa occurs in Addison's disease (Fig. 95) and of the skin during pregnancy. It also develops in large quantities in some tumors. Melanin pigmentation occurs in the oral cavity in the buccal mucosa and the gingiva (melanosis gingivae) as physiologic pigmentation. It is especially common in those individuals having deeply pigmented skin. However, there is not necessarily a correlation between skin color and oral pigmentation.

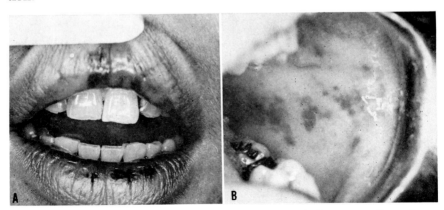

Figure 95. A, *Melanin pigment* of the lip in Addison's disease. B, Buccal mucosa of same patient.

BIBLIOGRAPHY

Fitzpatrick, T. B., Seiji, M., and McGregor, A. D.: Melanin pigmentation. New Eng. J. Med., *265*:328, 1961.

Freimer, E. H., and McCarty, M.: Rheumatic fever. Sci. Amer., *213*:66, 1965.

Gueft, B., and Ghidoni, J. J.: The site of formation and ultrastructure of amyloid. Amer. J. Path., *43*:837, 1963.

King, D. W.: Effect of injury on the cell. Fed. Proc., *21*:1143, 1962.

King, D. W., et al.: Cell death. Amer. J. Path., *35*:369, 1959.

Leevy, C. N.: Fatty liver and a review of the literature. Medicine (Balt.), *41*: 249, 1962.

Robinson, H. B. G., Boling, L. R., and Lischer, B. E.: in C. V. Cowdry: *Problems on Ageing*, 2nd ed. Baltimore, Williams & Wilkins Co., 1942.

Sokoloff, L.: The pathology of gout. Metabolism, *6*:230, 1957.

Spain, D. M.: Atherosclerosis. Sci. Amer., *215*:48, 1966.

Stamler, J.: Cardiovascular diseases in the United States. Amer. J. Cardiol., *10*:319, 1962.

Chapter 7
NUTRITIONAL DISTURBANCES

DEFICIENCIES OF BASIC FOODS

Malnutrition refers to a deficiency in the intake, digestion, absorption, and/or utilization of food. It readily can be seen that nutrition means more than mere diet. Food is necessary to supply energy to effect movement, growth, heat, repair, and other vital living processes. These processes of living cells constitute *metabolism*, which supplies the energy and nutrients for the formation and maintenance of cells. Since all body cells must rebuild or replace themselves from time to time, catabolic processes and anabolic processes are essential mechanisms of cells. Catabolic processes involve oxidation by which energy is released; anabolic processes involve a synthesis of complex cellular constituents from relatively simple raw materials (metabolites). Together the destructive (catabolism) and constructive (anabolism) processes constitute metabolism. Deficiency states may arise owing to interference with the energy mechanisms involved in metabolism or because of a deficiency in the quality or quantity of metabolites. A deficient intake of food may be associated with starvation, dietary fads, endemic food deficiencies, and inability to eat because of disease. The digestion of food may be interfered with by disease of the gastrointestinal tract, such as pancreatic disease, diarrhea, and cancer. Systemic metabolic disturbances may involve a defect in the metabolism of carbohydrates, proteins, and fat.

Fortunately there is a capacity, especially in animals, to adapt to a low intake or a deficiency of certain foods, viz., some animals can synthesize vitamin C. Humans may live adequately and indefinitely on 15 mg. of ascorbic acid, even though much larger amounts are considered normal for maintenance. Because of adaptive capacities, in order to produce deficiency manifestations, many of the "so-called" deficiency studies in reality are deprivation studies and are incompatible with life. The clinical application of the results of such studies is difficult, if not impossible.

It is important in considering the general properties of a diet, such

153

as carbohydrates, fats, proteins, and vitamins, to keep in mind that individuals vary considerably in their requirements. It is possible to receive toxic doses of vitamins A and D. Excessive amounts of vitamin A lead to the disease for which vitamin A normally would be used for treatment. Excessive vitamin D leads to calcific deposits, especially in the lungs. There is a tendency for diet and nutrition to go together, i.e., there is a direct correlation between diet and nutrition in a reasonably healthy individual. In a patient with systemic disease, there is a possibility that inadequate nutrition occurs directly because of the disease even with an adequate diet, although an inadequate diet also may be a contributory factor.

The effects of nutritional deficiencies are much more important in infants and growing children than in adults (including the growing and developing periodontal structures). The period at which the deficiency occurs is another factor that must be considered in evaluating studies of nutritional deficiencies.

Carbohydrates

Carbohydrates supply most of the energy which is essential to the living cells. Sugars and starches are examples of carbohydrates, and their digestion and utilization provide most of the caloric energy for metabolism. Glucose is a form of sugar found in the blood, much of which enters the liver through the hepatic portal vein. Glycogen is a complex carbohydrate synthesized from glucose by liver, muscles, and other tissues. Glycogen does not dissolve readily in water; consequently is an ideal storage material which can be used as it is needed by the tissues. When there is insufficient glucose in the blood, the condition is called *hypoglycemia,* which may be encountered when excessive amounts of insulin are administered to diabetic patients or when there is an excessive elaboration of insulin from a functioning tumor of the islet cells of the pancreas. A rather rare disorder of carbohydrate metabolism occurs in glycogen storage disease. In this disease there is an abnormal deposition of glycogen in liver, kidneys, and heart where it cannot be mobilized because of the absence of an enzyme in the liver and kidneys.

Fats

Lipids include all of the fat, oil, and fat-like substances which have a greasy texture and are relatively insoluble in water. Fat is an important source of calories, and an adequate caloric intake may not be possible without fat in the diet. Fat is also a necessary vehicle for the fat-soluble vitamins A, D, K, and E. A deficient lipid intake is encountered in starvation, in bizarre diets, and in some rather uncommon diseases with associated metabolic disorders characterized by lack of absorption of lipids from the gut. Where there is a dietary deficiency of lipids, there usually is an associated deficiency of protein, carbohydrate, and vitamin intake. Stored fats represent an important source of reserve energy for use when the metabolic needs of tissues are not met by dietary intake. In severe malnutrition, the catabolism of proteins takes place when the stored fat has been depleted.

Proteins

Proteins are necessary for growth and maintenance of body tissues, formation of antibodies, and maintenance of normal levels of serum protein. Proteins constitute a most important supporting structure of protoplasm and provide for a large variety of chemical reactions which are essential for life processes. Proteins can be broken down into simpler components called amino acids. Amino acids synthesized within the cells are called nonessential amino acids and are not needed in the diet, although they can be utilized if available. The amino acids not produced by the cells are called essential amino acids and thus are dietary essentials for man. Although there are over 20 amino acids, only eight are essential inasmuch as the rest may be synthesized by the cells. Since the proteins of every animal differ from those of every other animal, including man, it is impossible to transplant the organs of an animal to man because of the difference in proteins.

A deficiency of protein intake results in a loss of calories and a deficiency of essential amino acids, minerals, and lipotropic agents. Individuals with inadequate protein diets exhibit impaired wound healing, susceptibility to bacterial infection, and liver disease. The normal healthy adult should be in a state of nitrogen equilibrium (nitrogen intake equals nitrogen excretion). Negative nitrogen balance occurs in all diseases in which the destruction of tissue exceeds that of construction. A decrease in serum proteins may be encountered in liver disease or in association with an inadequate absorption of protein owing to starvation or intestinal disease. Some effects of general protein deficiencies have been derived from war records and studies of individuals in poverty. Other findings have been derived from hospitalized patients and animal studies (mostly where animals were completely deprived of protein).

One of the first clinical manifestations of general protein deficiency is edema and is called war and/or hunger edema. The permeability of the capillaries and the osmotic pressure are altered to the extent that fluid accumulates in the tissues. In such instances, no specific periodontal changes have been found in humans. In growing animals there is a decreased density of the periodontal membrane and new bone formation is inhibited, although eruption of the teeth continues. Adult animals do not show the periodontal widening in spite of the fact that collagen turnover is slow. Although proteins are essential for the animal to grow, periodontal pockets do not form from protein deprivation unless local factors are present. For changes to occur in the periodontium of an adult animal, the state of deficiency must be so severe that the animal is no longer capable of being on its feet. Even then, the animal dies before significant changes occur in the periodontium. In the growing animal, protein is essential for regeneration of collagen fibers and for building and maintaining the periodontal structures. In effect, deprivative changes represent inhibition rather than destructive changes.

DEFICIENCIES OF VITAMINS

Vitamins are relatively simple organic compounds necessary for normal function of the body. They are not synthesized in the body and must be obtained from the diet. Diseases due to vitamin deficiencies rarely exist in pure form, i.e., a deficiency disease is seldom due to a single vitamin. The clinical manifestations of diseases such as beriberi and pellagra are not eliminated by the therapeutic use of the constituents of the vitamin B complex considered to be the cause of the diseases, but require the use of the total complex of B vitamins to eliminate all the manifestations of these diseases. Also, the clinical symptoms of magenta tongue and angular cheilosis are primarily caused by a deficiency of riboflavin, but whole vitamin B-complex therapy is required, as well as other elements of adequate nutrition, for effective treatment.

There is no reason to believe that any beneficial results occur once the optimal level has been reached. Unfortunately, because of the absence of standard laboratory procedures to determine deficiencies, many unwarranted claims pertaining to so-called "subclinical deficiencies" have been made leading to the promiscuous use of vitamins. Conversely, many exaggerated claims have stimulated extensive use of vitamins. Such claims have led to many unjustifiable conclusions such as: vitamin C is of value in the treatment of simple gingivitis; vitamin A can prevent or cure the common cold in a well-fed individual; vitamin B is of value in the treatment of heart disease even when no deficiency exists; and vitamin B_{12} is of value in the treatment of osteoarthritis and nervous disease other than that associated with pernicious anemia. Such unfounded conclusions do not void the necessity for the proper use of vitamins in infants, growing children, pregnant women, and for diseases such as chronic gastrointestinal disturbances when vitamin, protein, or other deficiencies occur.

Vitamin A

Vitamin A is a fat-soluble substance found in fats, fish oils, carrots, green leaves, spinach, butter, milk, and egg yolks. It is essential to the proper maturation and maintenance of epithelial cells and for the production and maintenance of the visual purple in the retina. A deficiency of vitamin A (avitaminosis A) results in metaplasia or hyperkeratinization of the epithelium of hair follicles and other specialized epithelium, such as cornea, bronchi, kidneys, and salivary glands. The epithelial changes result in decreased resistance to infection because of the loss of cilia in the respiratory tract and a decrease in the secretion of the mucous glands of the conjunctiva. Changes in the developing ameloblasts have been reported but have not been confirmed in humans. The most commonly accepted signs of a deficiency of vitamin A are night blindness (nyctalopia), dry scaly skin, and dryness of the eyes (xerophthalmia).

In some diseases there is a decreased amount of vitamin A available. In cirrhosis of the liver there is very little vitamin A present. In both pernicious anemia and hyperthyroidism the level of vitamin A in the blood is diminished. It may also be deficient in obstructive jaundice, pancreatic disease, sprue, chronic diarrhea, and disorders of fat metabolism. Since fat probably is essential for the absorption of vitamin A or its precursors and bile is necessary for fat digestion and absorption, disturbances involving these processes may lead to a deficiency of vitamin A. Also vitamin A is probably stored in the liver, thus diseases of the liver might be expected to lead to vitamin A deficiency. A deficiency of vitamin A may develop under physiologic conditions when the demand is great as in periods of rapid growth.

Although malformation of bones may occur as a result of decreased endochondral bone formation in vitamin A deficiency, there is little evidence to suggest that a deficiency of vitamin A is significant in the etiology of periodontal disease in humans. Vitamin A is generally given to infants, growing children, pregnant women, and individuals with dietary deficiencies, hyperthyroidism, or diabetes mellitus.

Vitamin B Complex

The B vitamins are a group of substances somewhat related in function but not in chemical structure. They are often found together in foodstuffs. They may be divided into two groups: (1) those having to do with the formation of red blood cells, and (2) those concerned with the release of energy from food. Folic acid and B_{12} belong to the first group; nicotinamide, thiamin (B_1), and riboflavin (B_2) belong to the second group. All these vitamins, to some degree, may fall into both groups. Other members of the B-complex group include pantothenic acid, biotin, and para-amino-benzoic acid.

VITAMIN B_1.   Vitamin B_1 (thiamin hydrochloride) is water soluble and is found in yeast, egg yolk, bran, liver, and oysters. A deficiency of thiamin results in an accumulation of pyruvic and lactic acids in the tissues which causes impairment of cardiovascular, nervous, and gastrointestinal systems. The deficiency state is called *beriberi*. The manifestations of a deficiency of this vitamin include anorexia (loss of appetite), polyneuritis, gastrointestinal disturbances, edema, and cardiac failure. Beriberi is found chiefly in the Orient, where polished rice is the chief staple of the diet; however, sporadic cases occur in the southern states in this country. There is no established relationship between a deficiency of this vitamin and dental or periodontal disease.

VITAMIN B_2.   Vitamin B_2 (riboflavin) is a water-soluble substance found in yeast, liver, carrots, eggs, beef, cheese, and spinach. It is apparently important in the oxidative processes of the cell. A deficiency of riboflavin may result in glossitis, cheilosis, dermatitis, magenta tongue, or fissuring of the angles of the mouth. Frequently there is a scaly dermatitis around the ala of the nose. Fissuring of the angles of the mouth commonly is due to causes other than vitamin deficiencies (Fig. 96). Most fissuring at the angles of the mouth is probably due to accentuation of the nasolabial and commissural folds coupled with drooling, constant licking, poor hygiene, and, possibly, an overgrowth of monilia. With widespread, prolonged use of antibiotics an overgrowth of yeast organisms is a distinct possibility. A loss of filiform papillae and hyperplasia of the fungiform papillae may occur with burning sensations of the tongue and a deep magenta color (magenta tongue). There is no evidence to support a relationship between periodontal disease and a deficiency of this vitamin in humans. Laboratory studies in animals, which suggest a loss of alveolar bone, are deprivation studies, not deficiency studies, and cannot be extrapolated to periodontal disease in man. A deficiency of vitamin B_2 usually is associated with the inadequate consumption of meat, milk, and other proteins, but may be related to alcoholism, liver disease, and some forms of diarrhea.

NICOTINIC ACID.   Nicotinic acid (niacin) is found in yeast, eggs, milk, and fresh vegetables. It is water soluble and is necessary to catalyze certain oxidative processes of the cell. A deficiency of nico-

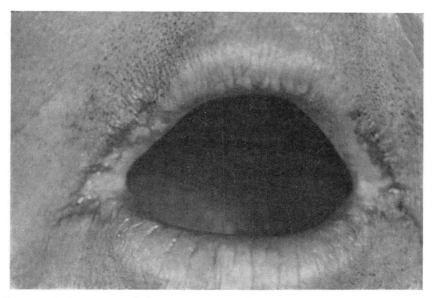

Figure 96. *Vitamin B deficiency.* Angular cheilitis of the type seen in severe riboflavin deficiency.

tinic acid causes pellagra. As is true of other deficiencies of B vitamins, *pellagra* usually accompanies poverty, chronic alcoholism, dietary fads, pregnancy, and chronic debilitating diseases. In advanced stages, dermatitis, diarrhea, and dementia are prominent features. The dermatitis involves sun-exposed surfaces. Early symptoms include a painful burning sensation of the tongue with later superficial painful tongue excoriations. Loss of papillae (atrophic glossitis) may be associated with vitamin B-complex deficiencies and other nutritional defects (Fig. 97). In general, the tongue is smooth, beefy-red in color, and sore. Although a deficiency of this vitamin has been considered as partly responsible for Vincent's infection because of the coexistence of Vincent's disease and vitamin B deficiency, no correlation has been demonstrated. In animals, ulceration and necrosis of the gingiva and leukopenia occur in terminal stages of nicotinic acid deprivation; however, a deficiency of nicotinic acid is not responsible for periodontal disease in humans. Pellagra is not considered simply to be due to a deficiency of niacin but also a deficiency of vitamin B_6 and other members of the B complex. The disease usually occurs in the spring and early summer because of the accumulated dietary deficiencies in the winter months associated with a large intake of corn, which apparently contains an antagonist to nicotinic acid.

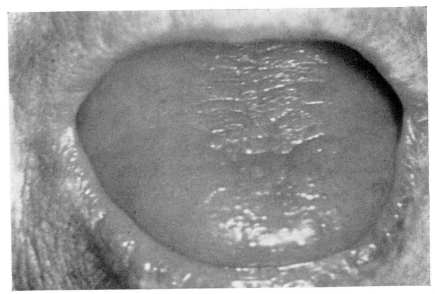

Figure 97. *Vitamin B deficiency.* The smooth, dark red tongue is typical of the change seen in pellagra as a part of niacin deficiency.

VITAMIN B$_6$.   Vitamin B$_6$ (pyridoxine) is found in yeast, cod liver oil, and corn. It functions as a coenzyme for several enzyme systems in amino acid metabolism. It is used prophylactically in tuberculous patients on prolonged isoniazid therapy. A deficiency results in convulsive seizures (in infants), anemia, and cardiovascular disturbances. Tongue lesions have been reported but not confirmed. It is of no significance in periodontal disease.

FOLIC ACID.   Folic acid (pteryoglutamic acid) is a combination of glutamic acid, pteridine, and para-aminobenzoic acid. It has an effect on hematopoiesis and has been used in the treatment of pernicious anemia; however, without the use of vitamin B$_{12}$, the neurologic symptoms remain unchanged. It is useful in the treatment of megaloblastic anemias of pregnancy and infancy, sprue, and anemia due to the folic acid antagonist aminopterin. Folic acid corrects glossitis (Fig. 98), diarrhea, and hemopoietic abnormalities in man. It is of no known significance in periodontal disease.

VITAMIN B$_{12}$.   Vitamin B$_{12}$ (cyanocobalamine) is found in liver, milk, and cheese and is essential for the maturation of red blood cells (erythrocyte-maturing factor). An intrinsic gastric factor is necessary for the absorption of this vitamin. It is almost ineffective when given by mouth if the intrinsic gastric factor is absent, but is very effective when injected intramuscularly. A deficiency results

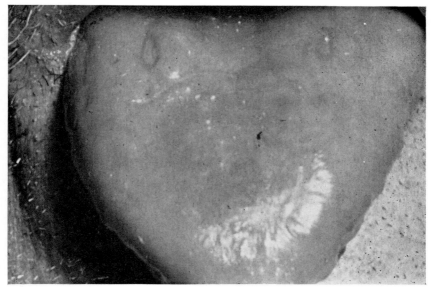

Figure 98. *Vitamin B deficiency.* A smooth atrophic pale tongue with super-ficial chronic ulcers is the type of change seen in severe deficiencies of riboflavin. A smooth tongue of this type is also seen in folic acid and B₁₂ deficiencies.

in a nutritional type of macrocytic (megaloblastic) anemia called pernicious anemia (p. 283). There is no established relationship between a deficiency of this vitamin and periodontal disease.

Vitamin C

Vitamin C (ascorbic acid) is found in citrus fruits, tomatoes, cabbages, and leafy green vegetables. It is essential in man for the formation of intercellular material in collagen, osteoid tissue, and dentin. A deficiency of this vitamin during growth accentuates the resulting defect. The manifestations of a deficiency of vitamin C is called *scurvy*. There is weakness, muscular pains, anemia, petechial hemorrhage, and hemorrhage beneath the periosteum, especially around the joints. The oral manifestations are related to the periodontium and occur in severity in proportion to the oral hygiene and the existing periodontal disease. Periodontal changes in the presence of local irritants include: gingival bleeding (Fig. 99), increased mobility of teeth, and increased severity of existing chronic destructive periodontal disease.

A severe deficiency of vitamin C must be prolonged in order to develop even minor gingival changes if oral hygiene is reasonably good. The term "subclinical deficiency" is used by some to indicate

12

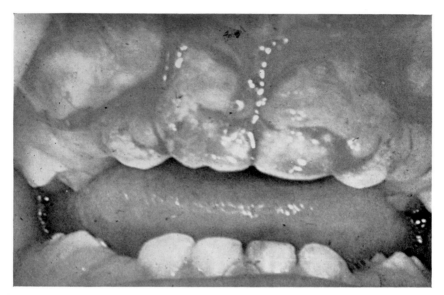

Figure 99. *Scurvy. Vitamin C deficiency in a young child.* Enlarged gingiva with extensive hemorrhage is the typical change of scorbutic gingivitis.

(1) a mild, anticipated deficiency of vitamin C without the usual manifestations of scurvy, except for what appears to be an increased tendency for gingival bleeding in the absence of easily seen local factors, or (2) an apparent increased bleeding tendency in the presence of gingivitis, which does not respond to local therapy because of a supposed mild deficiency in vitamin C. There has been no acceptable evidence to show that a subclinical deficiency of vitamin C is a factor in the cause of gingivitis or periodontitis. Studies have shown that scorbutic changes do not occur when the oral hygiene is good. In the presence of existing periodontal disease, scurvy will result in more severe periodontal disease because of decreased reparative ability, but a deficiency of vitamin C will not initiate periodontal disease. There is no acceptable evidence to show that the therapeutic use of vitamin C is valuable in the treatment of periodontal disease except when scurvy actually exists. Even then, vitamin C is not given to treat the periodontal disease, but to enhance the response of the tissues to the removal of irritating factors, such as calculus, that are the major causes of gingivitis or periodontitis.

Vitamin D

Vitamin D is found in fish oils, butter, milk, and eggs. It is necessary for the absorption of calcium from the gastrointestinal tract. Since vitamin D is related to the metabolism of calcium and phosphorus as well as to hormones, certain minerals, and other foods, investigations of a deficiency of vitamin D are complex. A deficiency of vitamin D and calcium and an altered calcium and phosphorus balance result in *rickets* in children and *osteomalacia* in adults. Rickets occurs in infancy and childhood owing to an inadequate intake of vitamin D or inadequate exposure to ultraviolet light (sunlight in which the ultraviolet rays are not blocked). Rickets is characterized by a failure of calcium salts to be deposited in the bones. The manifestations include a square-shaped head, bowing and deformities of the leg bones, and deformities of the sternum and costochondral junctions. Osteomalacia usually occurs as a result of an imbalance of calcium and phosphorus metabolism and is seen most commonly in starvation or with malnutrition, as occurs with sprue. Osteoporosis and deformities associated with fractures may occur. Changes in experimental animals include osteoporosis, reduction of the width of the periodontal membrane, osteoid tissue without calcification, and resorption of cementum. Variations of vitamin D, calcium, and phosphorus deficiencies produce similar periodontal changes. There is no increase in the prevalence or severity of chronic destructive periodontal disease or gingivitis in humans with rickets or osteomalacia.

Vitamin K

Vitamin K normally is formed in the intestinal tract by the action of microorganisms but is absorbed in the presence of bile. Vitamin K is essential for the synthesis of prothrombin in the liver. The prolonged use of antibiotics tends to inhibit the formation of vitamin K because of the antibiotics' effect on the intestinal flora. A deficiency of vitamin K results in defective clotting of the blood if prothrombin reserves in the liver are depleted. Vitamin K is of value in preventing hemorrhage when there is obstructive jaundice, pancreatic disease, or intestinal disturbances involving deficient bile production and malabsorption. The administration of vitamin K also is valuable for low prothrombin blood levels when anticoagulants are being used. Because vitamin K is not absorbed from the intestinal tract of the newborn for several days, the administration of the vitamin is of value in treating hemorrhagic disease of the newborn.

NUTRITION AND PERIODONTAL DISEASE

Although a well-balanced diet requires certain minimal amounts of each of the three basic foods—carbohydrates, fats, and proteins— the transformation of proteins into carbohydrates and fats makes the distinction between these basic foods less sharp than once thought. There is no absolute value for different foods, since requirements vary according to the needs of the individual. Pathologic changes secondary to malnutrition are variable. Combined deficiencies are the rule even in studies apparently designed to be pure deficiencies. For example, the patient with pellagra does not selectively eliminate only those foods containing niacin, but refuses to eat most foods and what is eaten is lost because of diarrhea, so the effect is generalized.

It is apparent, from experimental studies where animals have reached a terminus, that observations attributed to any single deficiency are most often pathologic changes brought about by multiple deficiencies and quite probably endocrine disturbances also. These observations point out the possibility of a wide variety of changes that may occur in the periodontium in deprived animals, especially when such conditioning or modifying factors as growth or local irritants are present.

The presence of osteoporosis, degeneration of the principal fibers, loss of alveolar bone support, and widening of the periodontal membrane cannot be considered as occurring in healthy individuals clinically; only in patients with severe deprivation states. More important, such changes do not represent chronic destructive periodontal disease with the presence of periodontal pockets. It is quite possible such changes can accelerate the progress of periodontal disease initiated by local factors, especially where deprivation is continued; however, any specific assessment as to degree of deficiency necessary to modify the progress of periodontal disease is purely hypothetical. Because of the adaptive capacity of most organisms and the absence of pure deprivation or the absence of such changes as are generally attributed to such states, it appears quite unlikely that clinical vitamin or protein deficiencies have any great bearing on the progress of periodontal disease. In such instances where the effect of a nutritional element is more specific to the periodontium, such as vitamin C, the progress of periodontal disease is accelerated and the tissues respond more unfavorably than normal to local irritants. Even so, there is no evidence to support the hypothesis that vitamin C is a significant factor in the progress of periodontal disease, unless the deficiency is absolute for long periods of time and other manifestations of scurvy are present.

From a practical clinical standpoint one might consider the nutritional status of a patient as having a bearing on periodontal disease when his clinical manifestations and history suggest the possibility. Clinical manifestations refer here to general manifestations; not a poor response to removal of local factors, unless all local irritants are definitely removed. Even with a nutritional disturbance, systemic treatment of periodontal disease is not the objective; the goal is the establishment of a good tissue response so that removal of local irritants will be most effective.

BIBLIOGRAPHY

Cannon, P. R.: *Some Pathologic Consequences of Protein and Amino Acid Deficiencies.* Springfield, Ill., Charles C Thomas, 1948.

Chawla, T. N., and Glickman, I.: Protein deprivation and the periodontal structures of the albino rat. Oral Surg., 4:578, 1951.

Dreizen, S.: Oral manifestations of nutritional anemias. Arch. Environ. Health, 5:66, 1962.

Mellanby, M.: Dental research with special reference to parodontal disease produced experimentally in animals. Dent. Pract., 59:227, 1939.

Ralli, E. P., and Sherry, S.: Adult scurvy and the metabolism of vitamin C. Medicine (Balt.), 20:251, 1941.

Russell, A. L.: International nutrition surveys: A summary of preliminary findings. J. Dent. Res., 42:232, 1963.

Snively, W. D.: The tiny giants. Bull. Path., 8:305, 1967.

Waerhaug, J.: Epidemiology of periodontal disease—review of the literature. In *World Workshop on Periodontal Disease.* S. P. Ramfjord, D. A. Kerr, and M. M. Ash, Eds. Ann Arbor, Mich., The University of Michigan Press, 1966.

Wolbach, S. B., and Bessey, O. A.: Tissue changes in vitamin deficiencies. Physiol. Rev., 22:233, 1942.

Wolbach, S. B., and Howe, P. R.: The incisor teeth of albino rats and guinea pigs in vitamin deficiency and repair. Amer. J. Path., 9:275, 1933.

Dental caries is a disease involving the hard portions of the teeth which are exposed in the oral cavity. It is characterized by the disintegration of enamel, dentin, and cementum forming open lesions (cavities). The process of disintegration is in part a demineralization and in part a dissolution of dental tissue. Dental decay or dental caries is the most common disease of the teeth. It is also one of the most common diseases found in man and occurs in all ages of both sexes in all the world's population. Although it is the most common chronic disease affecting man, dental decay is unique in that it cannot be repaired by the body. Less than 5 percent of the general population is immune to dental caries, but this immunity is an enigma to dental science. Because dental caries affects the health and economics of so great a portion of the population, it has great public health significance.

EPIDEMIOLOGY

Dental caries is primarily a disease of man, although it is found rarely in some animals. Dental decay in man involves all population groups, but the more primitive populations are less afflicted than people living in a more highly civilized society. Historical accounts of dental caries indicate that the disease is as old as recorded history and has increased in prevalence with the advancement of civilization. In studies of particular races of people and in comparison of primitive and civilized peoples, it has been demonstrated that caries incidence increases with the advancement of civilization and standards of living. In colonial times the incidence of caries was considerably lower than that presently found in the United States. It has also been shown that the incidence of dental decay has increased with the increased use of refined foods. Studies carried out on Eskimos living in native villages and not in contact with white man show that 1.2 percent of the teeth of these Eskimos are carious, whereas 18.1 percent of the teeth of those Ekimos living in an area where a trader sold some of the white man's foods were carious. Melanby observed the following effects of modern diet upon the incidence of caries in Rhodesia: about 5 percent of the adult natives who had had limited contact with a civilized diet exhibited caries; of the adolescents who had greater contact with a modern type of diet, 20 percent had caries; and of the children who had been exposed to modern foods for all their lives, 50 percent had dental caries.

Caries attack is evident as an individual reaches primary school age and remains high throughout the early teens. After the early teens the attack rate of caries declines slowly to about the age of 25 years when it drops off sharply. With advanced age carious activity may become highly active. Dental decay affects both sexes equally; however, the incidence may be higher in girls of school age because their teeth generally erupt earlier than boys, and, therefore, their teeth have a longer period of susceptibility to caries. Although some studies suggest racial differences in the incidence of dental decay, the suggested differences are probably due to variations in socioeconomic status rather than to actual racial susceptibility. That is, a higher incidence of dental decay might be expected in a socioeconomic strata where cariogenic foods, which are the least expensive, are widely used.

As previously mentioned, dental caries presents significant financial and public health problems. It is one of the most frequent causes of labor absenteeism in industry. It also ranked as the number one cause for rejection of draftees in World War II. It has been estimated that there are 500 million unfilled cavities in the United States in any given year. The American Dental Association estimated that 3.7 billion dollars was spent for dental services in 1967. Untreated carious teeth affect an individual's general health and may contribute to chronic debilitating diseases as well as to some fatal disease processes. Dental caries, therefore, presents one of the most important public health problems in the United States today.

ETIOLOGY

Some disease processes are produced by the introduction of specific organisms into the body, whereas other diseases are produced by a complex group of interrelated causative factors. Dental caries has a complex etiology, that is, its etiology is complicated by many indirect factors which obscure the direct cause or causes. Because of numerous indirect factors, the exact mechanism of caries attack is not positively established in all its details and, therefore, in part the etiology of caries is theoretical. The most universally accepted theory is the chemico-parasitic or acidogenic theory described by W. D. Miller in 1882. The chemico-parasitic theory proposes that carious lesions are the result of a process of demineralization of enamel and dentin by acids formed through bacterial enzymatic degeneration of carbohydrates and the proteolytic destruction of the organic portion of the enamel and dentin by the action of proteolytic microorganisms. With several factors being involved, it is understandable that the initiation and progress of dental caries are a complex process. The acidogenic theory of caries attack is based on the complex interrelationship of acids, plaques, microorganisms, carbohydrates and contributing or modifying factors.

Acids and Plaque

The protected surfaces of teeth that are not cleansed by the excursion of food develop a film or plaque of mucin precipitated from saliva. The plaque increases in thickness and extent by the entrapment of food debris and bacteria of various types. The plaque is firmly attached to the enamel or root surfaces of the tooth, and it is beneath these plaques that carious lesions are initiated. The organisms in the plaque produce enzymes which ferment carbohydrates, especially sugar and starch, to produce acid. The acid is held in contact with the tooth surface by the plaque and is protected from dilution by saliva by the thickness of the plaque. The concentration of the acid beneath the plaque increases when the supply of carbohydrate food is abundant and, therefore, causes rapid demineralization of the tooth. The rate of destruction depends upon the abundance of the plaque, the type and number of organisms present, the amount of carbohydrate available for conversion to acid, and the character (resistance) of the tooth surface. The process may be represented as follows:

$$\text{Carbohydrates} + \text{Enzymes} \longrightarrow \text{Acid}$$
$$\text{(Food)} \qquad \text{(Organisms)}$$

$$\text{Acid} + \text{Calcium} \longrightarrow \text{Demineralization}$$
$$\text{(Teeth)} \qquad \text{(Caries)}$$

Organisms of many varieties are normal inhabitants of the oral cavity and become incorporated into the plaque. Many are capable of producing acid by their action on fermentable carbohydrate food. Some not only produce acid but are able to survive in the acid medium which they create. This facility of bacteria to survive in an acid medium (aciduric bacteria) permits the development of a concentration of acid beneath the dental plaque high enough to cause demineralization. Acid production by organisms is rapid when there is an abundant carbohydrate substrate, but slow or nonexistent when it is not available. Acid production is also rapid when plaques are undisturbed, but interrupted when plaques are removed. The initiation of caries is, therefore, intermittent in character and is dependent on oral microorganisms, carbohydrates, acids, and modifying factors conducive to the production and adherence of the plaques.

Microorganisms

A large variety of cocci, bacilli, fungi, and other types of organisms constitute the normal flora of the oral cavity and demonstrate varying degrees of fermentive ability. Various forms of cocci and bacilli are capable of producing acid (acidogenic) and many are proteolytic, but of special significance are Lactobacilli. In addition to being capable of producing acid, Lactobacilli are able to survive in the high-acid media (aciduric) which they create. Lactobacilli have intense acidogenic properties and are constantly found associated with caries. Their constant association with caries and their intense ability to produce acid suggest that they are the most important organisms in caries production.

Carbohydrates

A substrate of carbohydrate upon which microorganisms act to produce acid is necessary to produce caries. It has been demonstrated that the most significant factors in the diet are refined sugars and starch, for whenever an isolated or primitive race is introduced to a "civilized" or refined diet of starches and sugars, the caries incidence increases. There is also a close correlation demonstrated between the dietary intake of sugar and caries activity. The presence of refined sugar in the diet has been shown to be the most important single dietary factor. The quantity, quality, and frequency with which carbohydrate is taken into the oral cavity determine the caries attack rate.

Modifying Factors

Modifying factors may considerably alter the attacking force to influence the location, extent, and activity of dental caries. The significant factors are dental plaques, the structure and resistance of teeth, the character of saliva, the position, form, and contour of teeth, oral hygiene, diet, and systemic factors.

DENTAL PLAQUES. The presence of dental plaques provides a habitat for the growth of organisms and retention of substrate and maintains the acid in contact with the surface of the tooth.

STRUCTURE AND RESISTANCE OF THE TEETH. The degree of calcification, the character of surfaces of the teeth and the resistance of the teeth do not determine whether or not the teeth will be attacked, but may determine the rate of attack. Surfaces that are poorly formed and irregular are conducive to the retention of plaques, whereas smooth, well-formed surfaces are less apt to retain plaques. Teeth that are highly calcified with complete maturation of the enamel are more readily destroyed by acid than those having poorly matured enamel with greater organic content. The enamel of some teeth may contain substances which are protective against caries activity, such as those containing fluorine.

SALIVA. It would seem reasonable to assume that if the saliva were acid in character caries activity would be high, and because of this assumption one often hears the statement that an individual with high caries activity has an acid mouth. However, saliva is naturally neutral and so buffered as to maintain the mouth at the neutral point even though acid is produced. Thus, the assumption that caries activity is related to an acid saliva is unfounded. However, the surfaces of the teeth beneath the plaque are at least partially separated from the buffering system of the saliva so that high concentrations of acid may occur. The physical character of the saliva, such as viscosity, has been suggested to be significant in dental caries because: (1) a thick mucinous saliva provides added material to form plaques, hangs to the surface of the teeth, and entraps food debris; and (2) conversely, a thin, copious saliva provides little material to form plaques and washes away food debris. It has been established that a marked decrease in the flow of saliva (xerostomia) predisposes to dental caries, however, small changes in the flow are probably of no significance. The salivas of people who are immune to caries have been extensively investigated to determine the presence of some specific buffer, antibacterial factor, or other protective mechanism but without success.

POSITION, SHAPE, AND CONTOUR OF TEETH. In situations where the teeth are malpositioned, there is a tendency for the retention of food debris and for plaques to be protected from the detergent action of food. Retention of debris about malpositioned teeth determines the point of attack and the rapidity of the progress of caries.

ORAL HYGIENE. If the mouth is self-cleansing, there is reason to believe that the caries attack rate is lower than when hygiene is poor. There is also much favorable evidence that the attack rate of caries can be altered by brushing the teeth immediately following the taking of food. By brushing the teeth immediately after eating, the plaques are disturbed and the substrate eliminated, thus reducing the attacking force. Unfortunately, most individuals do not effectively brush the interproximal surfaces of teeth which are the most prone to caries. Tooth-brushing has been especially effective in the control of cervical carious lesions which tend to occur beneath any materia alba retained on the surfaces of the teeth adjacent to the gingival margin.

DIET. The nature of the food eaten is significant in ways other than carbohydrate content. Soft diets have a tendency to adhere to tooth surfaces and have little detergent effect, whereas coarse diets have a detergent action and prevent the formation of plaques.

SYSTEMIC FACTORS. A natural immunity to dental caries suggests that something in the general physiology of an individual might be responsible for the lack of carious lesions, especially in view of the fact that Lactobacilli cannot be induced to live in the oral cavity of the naturally immune individual. Extensive investigation has been carried out to demonstrate such a systemic factor but without success.

CLINICAL ASPECT

When a caries attack rate is high and the process produces rapid destruction of the teeth, the process is said to be acute. When it involves nearly all surfaces of all teeth with rapid destruction, it is called *rampant caries*. If the process is slow, the destruction superficial, and only a few teeth involved, it is said to be *chronic*. If carious lesions recur about a previously treated lesion, it is designated *recurrent caries*. When the occlusal surface of a tooth is extensively destroyed or the proximal surface of a tooth and the surface is exposed to the cleansing excursion of food, the carious process may be markedly slowed or stopped; such lesions are designated *arrested caries*.

In the young child, dental caries is of an acute or rampant type, whereas in the adult it is of a chronic nature. Caries may be arrested in any age group, but most often chronic lesions are arrested. Rampant caries (Fig. 100) occur in the young and the very old. Recurrent caries occur at any age.

LOCATION OF CARIOUS LESIONS. Carious lesions are most often initiated in those areas of the teeth which are not self-cleansing and which are protected from the action of tooth-brushing. The most frequently involved areas are the pits and fissures, especially those of bicuspids and molars, which are often deep and sometimes poorly formed, viz., the enamel may not be fused at the depth of the fissure. The defective pits and fissures provide areas for the accumulation of plaques and the retention of food, so that the acid formed easily penetrates the tooth. When the carious lesion reaches the dentoenamel junction, it spreads laterally involving the under surface of the enamel and penetrating the dentin. This spread of the lesion beneath the enamel gives the impression that the lesion was initiated from within the tooth, an impression frequently expressed by lay

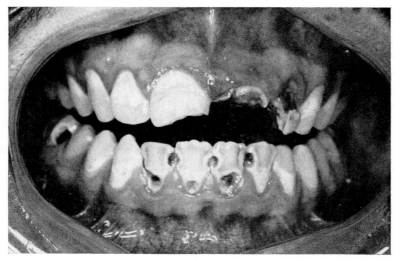

Figure 100. *Rampant dental caries.*

persons; there is, however, always a connection with the exterior, although it may be exceedingly narrow. Caries also occur in the buccal and lingual grooves of molars and the lingual pits of incisors. Pit and fissure caries occur as the initial attack sites in the majority of individuals and are of greatest incidence between eight and 16 years of age in permanent dentitions and between three and five years of age in deciduous dentitions.

The second most frequent location for caries is the interproximal area just beneath the contact point and is designated interproximal caries. Interproximal caries involve all teeth, but molars and bicuspids are involved more frequently than incisors. The maxillary incisors are more frequently involved interproximally than the mandibular incisors. Interproximal caries is of greatest incidence in permanent dentitions between 18 and 25 years of age, whereas in deciduous dentitions, it is between the ages of five and eight.

The third most common site of caries is the cervical region of teeth, especially when there is poor oral hygiene, gingival hyperplasia, and gingival recession. In permanent teeth, cervical decay usually occurs in individuals past the age of 35 years; it is rare in the deciduous dentition.

APPEARANCE OF CARIOUS LESIONS. The initial lesion of caries is a demineralization of the enamel, which reduces the index of refraction of the enamel causing the area involved to appear opaque and white (Fig. 116). This appearance is especially well demonstrated when demineralization occurs beneath the plaques at the cervical area of the teeth. After initial demineralization, the lesion becomes pigmented and discolored a light brown to black. The pigmentation is produced by the microorganisms present, by the liberation of the enamel pigment through disintegration of the enamel rods, and by the diffusion of pigmented substances present in the plaques. As the lesion develops the enamel is completely destroyed, producing a visible defect or cavity in the tooth surface which is white at its periphery where demineralization is slight and the surface is intact. The lesion becomes progressively darker in color toward its center where more structure is involved. As decalcification occurs the lesion becomes brown in color.

In the pits and fissures the center of the lesion is dark in color, while a large area around the fissure is opaque owing to the undermining of the borders. The enamel bordering the carious lesion is frequently fractured so that the border is irregular in shape and contour (Fig. 101). In extensive caries the lesion is a deep cavity with a pigmented base of soft, leathery dentin.

RADIOGRAPHIC FEATURES OF CARIES. X rays pass through the teeth in varying quantities depending upon the degree of calcification of the teeth. The quantity of x rays penetrating the tooth are registered on an x-ray film to produce a radiograph. Demineralized areas of teeth permit the passage of a greater quantity of x rays than normal tooth structure, so carious lesions are registered on the film as radiolucent (dark) zones. Occlusal caries is demonstrated as a widening of the developmental groove and a radiolucent area in the dentin beneath the fissure. Interproximal caries is recorded initially as a radiolucent spot on the mesial or distal aspect of a tooth just below the contact areas. In the more advanced lesion the area of enamel destruction is small, but the destruction in the underlying dentin is extensive. Cervical caries are not well demon-

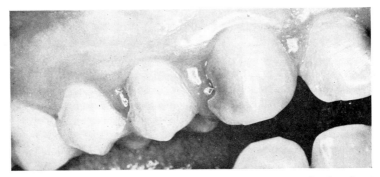

Figure 101. *Dental caries.* The gross defect with its irregular border is due to fracturing of unsupported enamel.

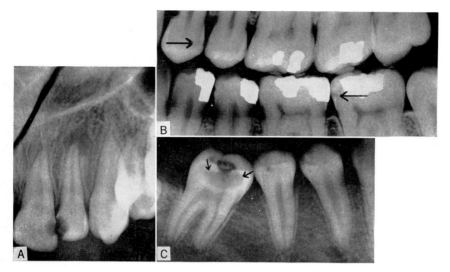

Figure 102. A, Mesial cavity in upper lateral incisor with periapical granuloma due to pulpal involvement. B, Interproximal caries indicated by arrows. C, Large undermining occlusal caries in first molar of a young person.

strated by x rays unless they are large. Recurrent caries may not be demonstrated by x ray unless it extends beyond the dental restoration. Radiographs are valuable for demonstrating the caries process and are used extensively in diagnosis to determine its presence (Fig. 102).

PATHOLOGY

PIT AND FISSURE CARIES. The caries process in developmental pits and fissures or grooves begins with the development of a plaque and the retention of food. The acid formed involves the interrod substance and penetrates along the enamel rods. Owing to the destruction of interrod substance, the enamel rods appear more prominent and cross striations are accentuated. There is also an accentuation of the lines of Retzius. The enamel rods radiate from the bottom of the developmental groove to the dento-enamel junction, and, thus, demineralization spreads along the enamel rods producing a pyramid-shaped lesion with the apex at the bottom of the groove and the base at the dento-enamel junction. In some instances, the enamel is incomplete at the base of the fissure and the dentin is attacked early; in other instances, the enamel is thick and the process is more advanced before the dentin is involved. As the carious process reaches the dento-enamel junction, it spreads along the junction beyond the area of initial penetration. The caries process involves the dentinal tubules and produces a pyramid-shaped lesion with its base at the dento-enamel junction and its apex toward the pulp (Fig. 103). When the lesion spreads along the dento-enamel junction, it produces demineralization from the dentin surface outward. By this time the enamel rods bordering the groove have been entirely demineralized, and the undermined enamel is easily fractured to produce a large cavity.

Smooth surface caries is essentially the same as pit and fissure caries except that the area of cavitation does not enlarge as rapidly as in pit and fissure caries. A lesion on a smooth surface (mesial and distal surfaces) is cone-shaped with the apex of the cone at the enamel surface. When the lesion reaches the dento-enamel junction, it spreads along the junction and penetrates the dentinal tubules

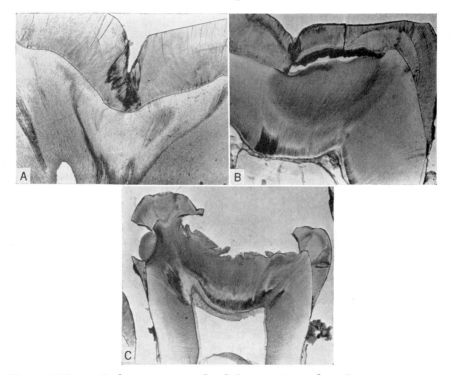

Figure 103. A, *Early caries in occlusal fissure of a molar.* Carious extension along dento-enamel junction and into the dentin is evident. B, *Caries of occlusal fissure* with backward caries and undermining of the enamel. Note extensive caries of dentin. C, *Extensive occlusal caries* with loss of enamel and dentin. Note early interproximal caries on right and advanced interproximal caries with loss of tooth substance on left side.

toward the pulp. Because of the configuration of the tubules, the carious lesion in the dentin progresses apically in a cone-shape with the apex toward the pulp (Fig. 104). Cavitation occurs as the result of complete destruction of the enamel rods and also as the result of the undermining of the enamel.

CARIES OF DENTIN. When cavitation of the enamel has occurred and the carious lesion has reached the dento-enamel junction, organisms penetrate the dentinal tubules and decalcification of the dentin occurs. The organisms may penetrate the tubules for a long distance from the surface of the lesion. In the tubules they continue to produce acid as well as to carry out proteolytic activity. Dentin is not as highly calcified as enamel, and complete disintegration of the dentin, which has a relatively high content of organic substance compared to enamel, could not occur simply by acid alone. In addition to acidogenic bacteria that cause decalcification, proteolytic organisms are present that elaborate proteolytic enzymes which destroy the organic material of the tubules and the dentin matrix.

Organisms may produce localized widening of the tubules and extend the carious process laterally through the side branches of the tubules and produce destruction of dentin matrix in a leaf-like pattern at right angles to the direction of the dentinal tubules (Fig. 105). Organisms collect in the clefts and extend the proteolytic

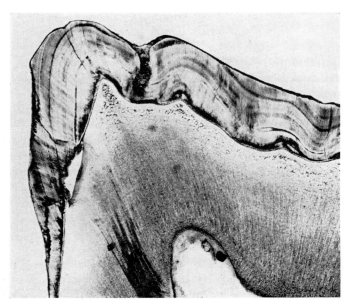

Figure 104. *Early interproximal caries.* Destruction of enamel and dentin at the dento-enamel junction.

13

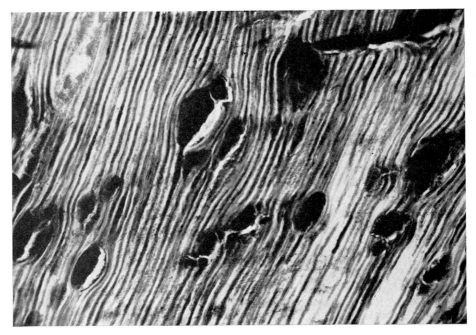

Figure 105. *Caries of dentin.* Large dark areas represent colonies of organisms in areas of destruction of dentin matrix.

destruction in all directions. The destruction of the dentin matrix results in cavitation of the dentin. Caries of dentin is, thus, a process of demineralization and proteolytic disintegration and depends on the action of two types of microorganisms.

CARIES OF THE CEMENTUM. This type of lesion occurs when recession of the gingiva exposes the cementum to the oral environment. Because of the more homogeneous, laminated character of the cementum, the carious process produces a smooth, saucer-shaped lesion. As in the dentin, caries of the cementum is a process of demineralization and proteolytic destruction. When the full thickness of the cementum is destroyed, the dentin is attacked the same as in other carious processes.

TREATMENT

The lesion of caries is unlike other areas of injury or damage in that there is no mechanism for repair. Therefore, the carious enamel and dentin must be removed and replaced with some type of filling material. The following steps are necessary for the proper restoration of carious teeth: all of the carious tissue must be removed to prevent recurrence beneath the restoration; the margins of the restorations must be sealed to prevent the penetration of caries along the boundary of the restoration; and the margins of the restoration must be placed on the surfaces of the teeth immune to caries.

SEQUELAE

When organisms invade the dentinal tubules, they destroy the dentinal fibers and progress toward the pulp. This process may result in the sclerosis of dentin, the formation of secondary dentin, or pulpitis.

Dental caries may stimulate the dental pulp to obliterate the dental tubules by depositing calcium salts in the dentinal fibers. The obliteration of the dentinal tubules reduces the porosity of the dentin and helps to delay the progress of caries by blocking the diffusion of acid and the ingress of organisms. The hypercalcified dentin is called sclerotic dentin or the translucent layer of Tomes.

The progress of caries may stimulate the odontoblasts to form additional dentin on the pulpal wall beneath the carious lesion. This additional or secondary dentin usually contains fewer tubules per unit area than primary dentin and so provides some reduction in the pathway for invasion of microorganisms. It also provides an additional bulk of material between the pulp and the carious lesion to protect against injury to the pulp.

If the carious process progresses more rapidly than sclerosis and/or secondary dentin formation, the pulp will be involved. Even before the dentin is completely destroyed, organisms and acid may reach the pulp and cause injury, which is manifest as the pain of a toothache. If the injury to the pulp is overwhelming, necrosis of the pulp occurs. When cavitation reaches the pulp, injury results and pulpitis is initiated. Pulpal disease is discussed in Chapter 9, page 184.

PREVENTION

In all disease processes prevention is a worthy aim; this is especially true of dental caries because the teeth are incapable of bringing about their own repair. One of the main objectives of dentistry is to prevent dental caries rather than to treat it. Much research has been carried out regarding the cause, the nature, the treatment, and the prevention of dental caries, but thus far this great effort has not provided the means for elimination of the disease. Research has provided some methods for the partial control and prevention of dental caries.

DIETARY CONTROL. Because caries attack is dependent upon the presence of carbohydrate foods in the diet, it is reasonable to believe that caries can be prevented by the control of carbohydrate foods in the diet. At the University of Michigan where the dietary control of dental caries has been studied by Bunting, Jay, and others, it was demonstrated that the rigid control of carbohydrate food in the diet for two weeks produced a significant reduction in the number of Lactobacilli present in the mouth and, thus, a reduction in caries activity. It was also demonstrated that after this initial period of rigid restriction of carbohydrate food, even though bread and potatoes (not sugar) were eaten, the Lactobacillus count remained significantly low in over 80 percent of the individuals following the diet. Furthermore, it was found that, if sugar were permitted at one meal per day for another period of two weeks, 70 percent of the individuals following the diet had a significantly low Lactobacillus count. Even after these patients were permitted to return to their regular diets which were high in sugar, their Lactobacillus count remained low for months to years, and caries activity was inhibited. By repeated checks for Lactobacilli a proper caries-inhibiting diet can be developed for almost every individual. Although the dietary control of dental caries is effective and satisfactory for individuals, it has to be carried out on a voluntary basis and for this reason is not applicable to mass populations.

DENTIFRICE CONTROL. Present-day advertising suggests or implies that numerous dentifrices are effective in the prevention of dental caries. This information is misleading although the use of a dentifrice would appear to be a possible and desirable means of caries prevention. Theoretically, a dentifrice might prevent caries by destroying the microorganisms responsible for producing acids; by blocking the enzymes produced by the Lactobacilli, so that they could not act on carbohydrates to produce acid; or by neutralizing the acids responsible for demineralization as they form. Such methods utilizing dentifrices have been investigated with varying degrees of effectiveness. The brushing of teeth with a penicillin dentifrice has been extensively investigated by Hill, Zander, and others. These investigators report some degree of effectiveness but not a successful means of control, because the organisms became penicillin-resistant and the patients became penicillin-sensitive. The use of enzyme-blocking agents has enjoyed a limited degree of success. Kerr and Kesel indicated a reduction in the caries rate by the use of an ammoniated dentifrice to neutralize the acid before it could act as an attacking force. The results of this study are highly questionable, and there is a lack of positive evidence that this is an effective means of caries control.

Recently, a large number of dentifrices containing fluorides have been introduced. Considerable variation has been reported in their effectiveness, in part owing to differences in fluoride activity present in the various dentifrices. All studies have shown some degree of caries control. It has been suggested that fluoride dentifrices are more effective after the topical application of fluorides. However, there is general agreement that fluoridation of communal water is the most effective method for the control of caries.

FLUORINE. As the results of observations that mottled enamel was produced by fluorine in drinking water and that patients having mottled enamel were somewhat immune to dental caries, it was suggested that fluorine, either applied to the tooth surface or incorporated in the drinking water, might provide a means of caries prevention. Extensive studies have been carried out on both the effect of topical application of fluorine and its addition to public drinking water. The topical application of 2 percent sodium fluoride to the surfaces of the teeth provides a reduction in dental caries activity. There is some disagreement as to the degree of effectiveness of this method of caries control. The usual procedure is to apply fluorine to the surfaces of the teeth after they have been well polished and dried. This is done at two and one-half, six, ten, and 16 years of age so that teeth are treated soon after they erupt. The addition of fluorine to public water supplies seems to provide the greatest protection and has the advantage of being an involuntary procedure which affects large population groups. The addition of 1 ppm of fluorine to drinking water provides a degree of protection against caries, but is not of sufficient concentration to produce mottling of the enamel. Fluoridation of communal water supplies presents a means of effectively controlling caries in a mass population. In spite of the benefits demonstrated by this method, strenuous objections have been raised by minority groups on the grounds that fluorides produce systemic toxic effects. There is no evidence that quantities of fluoride even several times 1 ppm have any general deleterious effects. The dental profession should vigorously support all measures to bring about fluoridation of communal water supplies.

BIBLIOGRAPHY

Bibby, B. G., Gustafson, G., and Davies, G.: A critique of three theories of caries attack. Int. Dent. J., 8:685, 1958.

Hill, T. J.: The use of penicillin in dental caries control. J. Dent. Res., 27: 259, 1948.

Hine, M. K.: Prophylaxis, toothbrushing, and home care of the mouth as caries control measures. In Dental Caries, Mechanisms and Present Control Technics as Evaluated at the University of Michigan Workshop. K. A. Easlick, Ed. St. Louis, C. V. Mosby Co., 1948.

Jay, P.: The role of sugar in the etiology of dental caries. J. Amer. Dent. Ass., 27:239, 1940.

Kerr, D. W., and Kesel, R. G.: Two-year caries control study utilizing oral hygiene and an ammoniated dentifrice. J. Amer. Dent. Ass., 42:180, 1951.

Koch, G.: Caries increment in school children during and two years after end of supervised rinsing of the mouth with sodium fluoride solution. Odont. Rev., 23:323, 1969.

Marshall-Day, C. D., and Sedwick, H. J.: Studies on the incidence of dental caries. Dent. Cosmos, 77:442, 1935.

Mellanby, M.: Effect of diet on the resistance of teeth to caries. Proc. Roy. Soc. Med., 16:74, pt. 3, 1923.

Miller, W. D.: *Microörganisms of the Human Mouth*. Philadelphia, S. S. White, 1890.

The 1968 Survey of Dental Practice. American Dental Association, Chicago, 1968.

Shaw, J., Ed.: Fluoridation as a public health measure. American Association for Advancement of Science, Washington, D.C., 1954.

Socransky, S. S.: Caries-susceptibility tests. Ann. N.Y. Acad. Sci., 153:137, 1968.

Whipple, H. E., Ed.: Mechanisms of dental caries. Ann. N.Y. Acad. Sci., 131: 685, 1965.

Zander, H. A., and Bibby, B. G.: Penicillin and caries activity. J. Dent. Res., 26:365, 1947.

Chapter 9
DENTAL PULP
DISEASE

Dental pulp is the soft tissue portion of a tooth and contains the tooth's blood vessels and nerves. The pulp is the formative organ for the dentin and reacts to environmental stimuli in a protective manner by producing sclerotic and secondary dentin. The dental pulp is a delicate type of connective tissue which is protected by being completely surrounded by dentin. In spite of its protection, the pulp is subject to injury by thermal changes, by invasion of microorganisms through advanced carious lesions, and by mechanical trauma, such as is produced by traumatic occlusion or a physical blow. The most frequent response of the pulp to injury is inflammation and is designated pulpitis.

The normal pulp is a delicate mesenchymal tissue composed of delicate connective tissue fibers loosely arranged and separated by intercellular fluid. It contains numerous blood vessels having unusually thin walls and delicate nerve fibers which react to all noxious stimuli as pain. The periphery of the pulp is surrounded by a single layer of columnar cells responsible for dentin formation and called odontoblasts. They form dentin starting at the enamel or cemental surface and migrating inward. This process is a continuous one throughout life and results in a continual reduction in size of the pulp chamber. As the pulp chamber becomes smaller with age, the pulpal tissue becomes more compact and loses some of its ability to react favorably to injury. Associated with this decreased ability to react to injury, there usually is a deposition of calcium salts into the pulp tissue, so that pulpal calcification is a constant finding in the teeth of old people.

ETIOLOGY

Inflammation of the dental pulp may be produced when it is invaded by organisms through a deep carious lesion. When a deep carious area is restored by a metallic restoration without placing an insulating substance in the base of the cavity, the pulp is subjected to frequent and wide ranges of temperature change because the metal of the restoration is an excellent conductor of heat and cold. Severe changes in temperature may be transmitted to the pulp from eating something ice cold followed almost immediately by something very hot. The pulp may be subject to a sudden temperature change because of the heat generated in the preparation of a cavity or the polishing of a filling. The rapid and forceful preparation of cavities without coolants and the forceful and rapid polishing of restorations and teeth generate sufficient heat to produce pain. If the heat is prolonged or intense, permanent injury to the pulp results.

PULPITIS

Inflammation of the pulp occurs when it is injured. This inflammatory reaction to injury, pulpitis, is usually attended by pain and described by the patient as a toothache. Pain is a fairly constant symptom of pulpitis, but the presence of pain in the region of the teeth is not always indicative of pulpal disease. The character, intensity, and duration of a toothache are diagnostic symptoms dependent upon the type of pulpitis present. The pulpal reaction to injury depends on the nature of the injury, the degree of pulpal damage, and the vitality of the pulp. Pulpitis may be divided into the following types, depending upon the degree of involvement and the nature of the inflammatory response.

HYPEREMIA OF THE PULP. In the initial stage of pulpal inflammation there is a dilatation of blood vessels permitting more blood to be carried to the area of injury. This is designated hyperemia of the pulp and may be either on the arterial side of circulation (active hyperemia) or on the venous side of circulation (passive hyperemia). Active hyperemia is produced during the cutting of cavity preparations, the polishing of restorations, or the application of some other sudden mild stimulus. The active hyperemia results in pain which subsides rapidly as soon as the stimulus is removed. If active hyperemia is persistent, passive hyperemia will ensue, and, although the pain may not be so intense as in active hyperemia, it is of longer duration.

Regardless of the type of injury, the initial pulpal reaction is always manifest as hyperemia, which produces somewhat typical clinical symptoms. The tooth is uncomfortable and pain is produced by cold and relieved by heat. Hyperemia may persist for a long time due to mild stimuli and then regress when the stimuli are removed. However, it may be the initial phase of a severe inflammatory response resulting in severe pulpal damage. When hyperemia is the initial phase of an inflammatory response and is followed by exudation, the pulpal response is *simple pulpitis*.

SIMPLE PULPITIS. This process is an inflammatory response to

injury in which there is hyperemia and exudation. Owing to changes
in the vessel walls associated with dilatation, plasma and white
blood cells pass through the vessel walls into the tissue spaces (exudation). If only a portion of the pulp is involved, it is termed partial
simple pulpitis; if the entire pulp is involved, it is total simple pulpitis. Partial simple pulpitis is produced under a large filling that is
poorly insulated or as the result of a cavity which approximates the
pulp. It may be due to microorganisms invading the pulp through
a carious lesion.

The symptoms associated with pulpitis depend on the degree of
pulpal involvement. In partial pulpitis the pain is intermittent and
of slight degree. The pain is intensified by cold and relieved by heat.
As the involvement of the pulp becomes more extensive, the pain
becomes more intense, more frequent, and of longer duration, until
there is total involvement of the pulp when the pain becomes very
intense and continuous.

Partial simple pulpitis is a reversible process and the pulp usually
recovers with the elimination of the injurious agent. In total simple
pulpitis the pulp does not recover and the tooth must have a root
canal filling or be extracted. When simple pulpitis is due to microorganisms, pus may be formed; this type of pulpitis is called *suppurative pulpitis.*

Suppurative Pulpitis. Like simple pulpitis, suppurative pulpitis
may be partial or total. Suppuration may be limited to a small area
of the pulp. The focal accumulation of pus is designated a pulp
abscess. The entire pulp may become suppurative and the pulp
chamber fills with pus; this is designated total suppurative pulpitis.
The symptoms of suppurative pulpitis are severe. In partial suppurative pulpitis the symptoms may consist of an intermittent, sharp and
throbbing pain; however, if total suppurative pulpitis ensues, the
symptoms become more intense and continuous. The pain accompanying total suppurative pulpitis is said to be one of the most
severe pains experienced by man. As pus accumulates, there is an
increase in pressure within the pulp chamber due to both fluid and
gas. When heat is applied to an involved tooth the gas expands
in the pulp chamber and the pain is intensified; when cold is applied,
the gas contracts and the pain is relieved. Owing to the increased
pressure within the pulp chamber, some of the exudate is forced out
through the apical foramen initiating an inflammation in the periapical tissues which is discussed under sequelae of pulp disease.
Suppurative pulpitis, whether partial or total, is irreversible and
necessitates root canal therapy or extraction of the involved tooth.

Gangrenous Pulpitis. This pulpitis is an ischemic necrosis produced by alteration of the circulation of the pulp. It may result from

an intense hyperemia in which there is stasis of the blood and thrombosis. With pulp necrosis there is a production of gas producing the same symptoms and sequelae as suppurative pulpitis. Ischemic necrosis of the pulp may also be produced as the result of a blow which causes displacement of the apex and tearing of the vessels at the apex so that the pulp loses its blood supply. Pulp necrosis from this type of injury is usually not attended by pain because the continuity of the nerve is lost at the same time as the blood supply. The sequelae may be the same as those resulting from suppuration and from necrosis secondary to hyperemia and thrombosis.

ULCERATIVE PULPITIS. This type of pulp disease is due to exposure and injury of the pulp by caries. Ulcerative pulpitis usually does not produce symptoms except when a carious cavity is filled with food. Owing to the opening produced by extensive caries, the pulp is no longer encased in a closed chamber and pressure can no longer be built up in the pulp chamber due to hyperemia or accumulated exudate. It is for this reason that symptoms are produced only when the pulp is directly stimulated or the opening into the pulp is obstructed and an exudate accumulates. Ulcerative pulpitis is not reversible and must be treated by endodontics or extraction. In some instances, the exposed pulp may attempt to repair the exposed area by the accumulation of granulation tissue which is designated chronic productive pulpitis.

CHRONIC PRODUCTIVE PULPITIS. This condition occurs only in young teeth in which the pulp exhibits extreme vitality. It is seen most often in the first permanent molars of children eight to 12 years of age who have extensive and rapidly progressing carious lesions resulting in extensive destruction of the crown and wide exposure of the pulp (Fig. 106). In the area of exposure, granulation tissue is produced which herniates into and sometimes more than fills the cavity. At first the tissue is soft, red, and bleeds easily. Later it becomes the color of the buccal or gingival mucosa owing to epithelialization of the surface. The sharp margins of the cavity dislodge epithelial cells from the buccal mucosa or tongue that are transplanted onto the granulation tissue and grow to cover the entire mass. These polypoid masses are designated pulp polyps. They are insensitive to pressure and are, therefore, asymptomatic. The presence of a pulp polyp usually necessitates extraction of the tooth.

PULPAL CALCIFICATION. The deposition of calcium salts in the pulp is a constant finding with advancing age. Some degree of calcification is present in the pulps of all adults, but may be more marked in some individuals than others. The calcium salts are deposited in both coronal and radicular portions of the pulp. In the coronal part of the pulp, the calcium salts are deposited in circumferential layers

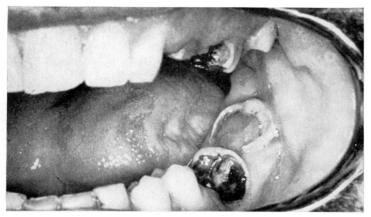

Figure 106. *Chronic hyperplastic pulpitis ("pulp polyp").* Large mass of granulation tissue filling extensive occlusal cavity of lower second molar.

about a central nidus and are called pulp stones or denticles. In the radicular part of the pulp, the calcium salts are deposited as fine granular particles along the path of the vessels and are designated linear calcification. Pulpal calcification indicates that some degree of involution of the pulp has taken place; however, it rarely produces symptoms even though almost the entire pulp may be calcified.

INTERNAL RESORPTION. Internal resorption is a process in which the dentin is resorbed by the pulp tissue and results in an increase in size of the pulp chamber even to the point of exposing the pulp when the full thickness of the dentin and enamel or cementum is resorbed. The process of resorption initially occurs more commonly in the midportion of the root but may gradually extend through the entire thickness of the root. Internal resorption occurs much less often in the coronal portion of the pulp than in the root portion. When the process of resorption extends to the enamel, the vascular tissue of the pulp shows through the translucent enamel and appears as a pink spot in the tooth. Internal resorption is probably initiated by pulpal injury as the process is frequently seen following pulpotomy (the amputation of the diseased portion of a pulp). Internal resorption usually arises near the amputation site; however, in most cases, injury is not evident. Symptoms of internal resorption are not present until the full thickness of the tooth is destroyed and the pulp is exposed. With the exposure of the pulp, the tooth must be extracted, as endodontic therapy is unsuccessful.

SEQUELAE

Pulpal disease, whether due to degeneration or infection, if untreated, produces disease processes in the periapical region or the surrounding jaw. During degeneration and necrosis of the pulp there is an increase in pressure within the pulp chamber forcing degradation products or the elements of infection through the apical foramen into the periapical zone. This incites an inflammatory response in the periapical tissues which may be localized to that area or spread into the contiguous tissues. Each of the changes so produced are discussed separately.

ACUTE PERIAPICAL INFLAMMATION (PERIAPICAL ABSCESS). In association with severe acute pulp disease such as suppurative pulpitis, gangrenous pulpitis, or complete pulpal degeneration, material from the pulp is forced into the periapical area and produces an acute inflammatory response (Fig. 107). Inflammation in the periapical areas produces pain and swelling of the periodontal tissues. The swelling causes the tooth to extrude slightly from the alveolus so that when the teeth are brought into occlusion, the extruded tooth contacts before the others. This premature contact forces the tooth

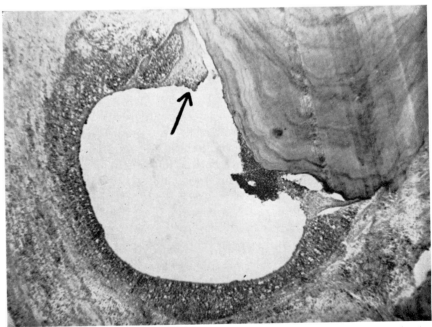

Figure 107. *Chronic periapical abscess.* The space adjacent to the root tip was filled with pus which was lost in preparation of the specimen. The border of the space is granulation tissue with early epithelial proliferation indicated by the arrow.

into the alveolus intensifying the pain. Patients refer to this situation as an "ulcerated tooth." Radiographs show a slight thickening of the periodontal membrane at the apex of the involved tooth.

PERIAPICAL GRANULOMA. A granuloma results when the inflammatory process at the apex is minimal and the body localizes the inflammation to the periapical zone. It is usually the result of partial, slow degeneration of the pulp. It may follow pulp death from a severe, sudden blow or with exposure of the pulp due to caries. Periapical granulomas also occur at the apex of improperly treated root canals. There is some destruction of periodontal membrane and alveolar bone with attempted repair and the formation of granulation tissue. The zone of reaction is usually small and sharply limited to the apical area which can be seen in the x-ray film as a radiolucent area localized to the apex of the root (Fig. 102). Periapical granuloma may persist for long periods of time without producing symptoms but without apparent cause may become acute.

RADICULAR CYSTS. These cysts arise in long-standing periapical granulomas when there are epithelial rests in the periapical area. The inflammatory process stimulates proliferation of the epithelial rests in the periapical area and, as they grow, surround the apex of

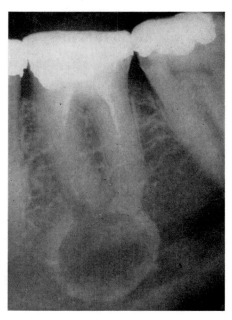

Figure 108. *Periapical cyst.* First molar with incomplete root canal filling. The periapical cyst is sharply demarcated by peripheral condensing osteitis.

the root or cover the surface of granulation tissue adjacent to the root. This results in an epithelial-lined space at the apex which is called a radicular cyst (Fig. 108). Like the granulomas, they remain present without symptoms for long periods of time. They gradually increase in size due to accumulation of fluid in the cyst space and produce destruction of the surrounding bone. In exceptional cases they may produce expansion of the jaw. Radicular cysts frequently undergo exacerbation of the inflammatory process and produce swelling and pain in the jaw.

CELLULITIS. Cellulitis is a diffuse inflammation of the soft tissues surrounding the jaws produced by the spread of an acute periapical inflammation outside the jaw. In some cases, the periapical inflammation is severe and the body is unable to localize it to the periapical area. The pus escapes into the surrounding tissues, especially facial spaces, resulting in marked swelling, intense pain, and general malaise with elevation of temperature. Cellulitis is a severe process which, if not given immediate attention, may kill the patient.

PARULIS, FISTULA, GUM BOIL. These terms are used to indicate the spontaneous drainage of a periapical abscess. In children the roots of the deciduous teeth are close to the surface of the jaw and the cortical bone is thin, so that periapical abscesses easily rupture to the exterior of the jaw. The pus accumulates beneath the mucosa producing a localized swelling which ruptures allowing pus to escape into the mouth. The elevated area with an opening from which pus escapes is called a parulis or gum boil (Fig. 109). Once drain-

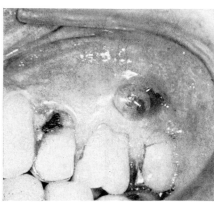 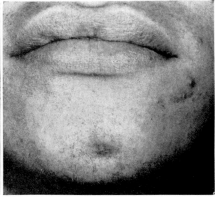

Figure 109. *Parulis or "gum boil."* Note nodular area on gingiva above first molar with draining sinus in center of the mass.

Figure 110. Draining sinus on the chin from area at apex of mandibular incisors.

age is established, symptoms subside and the drainage is persistent until the tooth is treated or extracted. On some occasions the pus makes its exit through the jaw apical to the mucobuccal fold and migrates through the tissue to the skin. It ruptures through the skin and the pus escapes to the exterior. The drainage tract is termed a fistula or sinus tract (Fig. 110). A draining sinus persists until the involved tooth is treated or extracted.

OSTEOMYELITIS. An inflammatory process of bone with the accumulation of pus in the marrow spaces is designated osteomyelitis. When pus from a periapical abscess cannot escape through the cortex of the jaw, it may spread in the marrow spaces and involve a large area of the jaw. Owing to accumulation of pus in the marrow spaces, the bone undergoes necrosis attended by pain and swelling of the area. The patient has malaise and an elevation of temperature. The dead bone acts as a foreign body and separates from the living bone, and it must be removed either by the body or by surgery. The dead bone, which is separated from the living bone, is designated a sequestrum and may be spontaneously evulsed from the jaw.

BIBLIOGRAPHY

Johnson, R. H., Christensen, G. I., Stifers, R. W., and Loswell, H. R.: Pulpal irritation due to the phosphoric acid component of silicate cement. Oral Surg., 29:447, 1970.
Zach, L., Topal, R., and Cohen, G.: Pulpal repair following operative procedures. Oral Surg., 28:587, 1969.

Chapter 10

STAINS AND ACCRETIONS

In the human mouth, the teeth and tongue tend to be unclean in spite of natural cleansing factors present which act to maintain a clean mouth. The cleansing action of saliva, detergent foods, tongue, cheeks, and lips, the smoothness of the surfaces of teeth, shallowness of gingival crevices, and functional arrangement of teeth, all tend to keep the mouth free from stains and accretions. Minor alterations in the smoothness of the teeth, deepened gingival crevices, indolent mastication, altered gingival form, lack of a detergent diet, loss of teeth, malocclusion, and other factors predispose the mouth to the deposition of stains and accretions. The natural factors of self-cleansing may not be able to eliminate contaminants such as the debris of soft food, tobacco, metallic salts, medicaments, and other factors which alter the normal chemical, bacterial, and physical balance of the forces of oral hygiene in the mouth. Unfortunately, with our present mode of living, the potential for uncleanliness usually far exceeds the natural ability of the mouth to maintain a state of cleanliness without assistance. This assistance is the responsibility of the patient, as well as the dentist and the hygienist, and requires some understanding of the nature of stains and accretions which deposit on the teeth. This understanding is necessary for the prevention of stains and accretions, for an understanding of the procedures to be used in their removal, and for an appreciation of the benefits of their removal.

The degree of malhygiene of the mouth varies from one individual to another. The variation depends upon the natural factors pertaining to oral hygiene as well as assisting factors, such as home care and prophylaxis. Many of the factors predisposing to uncleanliness are known and can be eliminated. However, many factors in oral hygiene, both natural and synthetic, remain to be determined. For example, little is known about the reason why calculus forms readily in one person's mouth and not in another's, nor how calculus can be prevented from forming subgingivally or in areas which cannot be reached effectively by home-care methods. However, it is well known that stains and accretions can be prevented where the cleaning action of the mouth is functioning normally and is assisted by proper home-care procedures. Thus, the best prevention of mal-hygiene at the present time is in the use of adequate home-care procedures and in establishing and maintaining the natural factors of cleanliness. Once the functional form of the teeth and gingiva have been altered by disease, the need for determined home care becomes even greater than before. Thus, although poor oral hygiene is the basic causative factor of periodontal disease, the effects of periodontal disease in altering normal factors of cleanliness are significant factors in the formation of stains and accretions.

PHYSIOLOGY OF ORAL HYGIENE

As already mentioned, certain factors predispose to the maintenance of a clean mouth. These factors are related to the form and function of gingiva and teeth, the arrangement of teeth, the saliva, bacterial flora, diet, and type of mastication. In order to understand the mechanism of malhygiene and some of the factors predisposing to its inception, it is necessary to consider these factors.

ARRANGEMENT OF THE TEETH. The teeth are arranged in the dental arches in such a manner as to provide adequate prehension, incision, and crushing of food and to protect the periodontium against impingement. The close approximation of the teeth with continuous interproximal contacts, the smooth transition of one surface of a tooth to another, and the presence of interdental papillae prevent the accumulation of food in the interproximal areas. This continuity also allows detergent foods and the action of the cheeks and tongue to cleanse the surfaces of the teeth. Any alteration of the continuity of the arches and interdental papillae, such as the loss of teeth or malposition of teeth, prevents the adequate cleansing of exposed interproximal surfaces and predisposes to the accumulation of stains and accretions.

FORM OF THE TEETH. The normal form of the teeth is important to the functions they perform in mastication and in the protection of the periodontium. Abnormalities of curvatures associated with either developmental disturbances or restorations may interfere with the normal cleansing action of the tongue and cheeks and the detergent action of coarse foods; this makes cleaning the teeth difficult even by home-care methods. Improper interproximal contacts, open contacts, poor marginal ridges, and flat lingual and buccal surfaces of teeth often lead to the impaction of food and the accumulation of debris in the region of the free gingival margin. Rough and porous surfaces predispose to the attachment and accumulation of stains, plaques, and accretions.

FORM OF THE GINGIVA. The form of the gingiva and its adaptation to the teeth are intimately related to the protection of the periodontium and to good oral hygiene. Hyperplasia of the gingiva, recession of the gingiva, deepening of the gingival crevices, and malposed teeth are significant factors in the accumulation of stains and accretions on the teeth. Hyperplastic gingival tissues are not closely adapted to the surfaces of the teeth; this alteration of gingival form allows stains and accretions to accumulate on the teeth adjacent to the altered gingival margins where the action of the tongue, cheeks, and toothbrush are not effective in their removal. When the gingiva is closely adapted to the surfaces of the teeth and the gingival crevice is shallow, the action of the cheeks and tongue, the action of detergent food, and the action of the toothbrush are able to maintain the surface of the tooth adjacent to the free gingival margin relatively free from stains and accretions.

SALIVA. The free flow of saliva is important to cleansing the teeth because of its washing action. Individuals with dry mouth (xerostomia) accumulate large quantities of accretions on their teeth. It is also probable that ptyalin, a starch enzyme present in the saliva, acts to digest residual starch particles left on the teeth. A lack of saliva also predisposes to the overgrowth of certain microorganisms that are important in the formation of soft plaques and calculus on the teeth.

MASTICATION. The character of a person's diet is also an important factor in the mechanical cleansing of teeth. Coarse, detergent foods tend to clean the surfaces of the teeth, whereas soft, sticky foods tend to adhere to the teeth. This difference may be readily appreciated if a coarse food such as celery is chewed after a soft food such as pie is eaten. The chewing action itself is important to the mechanical cleansing of teeth and its effect may be easily observed in the presence of unilateral mastication, wherein the individual usually does most chewing on on side of his mouth. This leads to an accumulation of food debris and accretions on the side which is not being used.

RESTORATIONS. Restorations with "overhanging margins" lead to the accumulation of plaques and accretions in areas which cannot be effectively cleaned by natural mechanisms or by home-care methods. Porous restorations with imperfectly adapted margins lead to the accumulation of pigments and stains which cannot be removed. Fixed bridges that are made without due consideration for access in cleaning inherently predispose to the accumulation of accretions.

STAINS

Staining of teeth may result from pigments or colored substances taken into the mouth, such as tobacco, medicines, dentifrices, foods, and from the action of chromogenic bacteria, or from the deposition of pigments in the structure of the tooth itself as the result of systemic disease or disease of the pulp. Stains derived from substances taken into the mouth and from chromogenic bacteria are designated *exogenous stains;* those derived from blood-borne pigments associated with systemic disease or as a result of disease of the pulp are designated *endogenous stains.* Exogenous stains may be further subdivided into those of *metallic* composition and those of *non-metallic* composition. Exogenous stains are deposited in films and plaques on teeth and in rough, pitted and porous surfaces of teeth. Exogenous staining of teeth is usually indicative of poor oral hygiene; endogenous staining is most often indicative of pulpal death.

Exogenous Stains

Metallic Stains. Metallic staining of teeth is generally associated with the occupational hazards of metal workers or with the use of medicines containing metals or their salts. Metallic dust, associated with the fabrication of metal products, may lead to inhalation and accumulation of metals in plaques and films present on the teeth. Thus, the degree of staining is related not only to the amount of exposure to the dust, but also to the degree of malhygiene which is present. Metals or their salts may penetrate pits, fissures, cracks, or hypocalcified areas of the teeth. They may penetrate porous filling materials or the margins of imperfectly adapted restorations. A *bluish-green* stain may occur on the surfaces of the teeth of workers in copper, brass, or bronze. This stain may be removed by polishing if it has not penetrated into the tooth structure. *Brown* stains may result from the use of drugs containing iron or from the industrial inhalation of iron-containing metals. The staining associated with iron-containing drugs is often more generally distributed throughout the mouth than that arising from the inhalation of metallic dusts. Iron stains may be brown to black and must be differentiated from tobacco stains. Individuals drinking water containing a large amount of iron may also incur brown stains on their teeth. *Silver* staining most often occurs as the result of the use of silver nitrate on the teeth by the dentist. This black stain is often present on the necks of the teeth and tends to penetrate deeply into the cementum and dentin. Application of silver nitrate to a cavity preparation often results in the penetration of the black-silver stain into the dental tubules giving the tooth a dark bluish-gray discoloration, especially if the application of silver nitrate has been extensive. Mercury and manganese give rise to black stains and nickel to green stains.

NONMETALLIC STAINS. Nonmetallic stains may be associated with the incorporation of pigmented substances into plaques and accretions on teeth, rough, pitted and decalcified surfaces of teeth, and remnants of the enamel cuticle. Stains involving the mucinous deposits and accretions on the teeth generally are easily removed with the accretions. Those associated with the enamel cuticle are more difficult to remove. It may be impossible to remove stains which have penetrated pits, fissures, and porous areas of teeth.

BLACK STAIN. Two variations of black stain of nonmetallic origin may occur on the teeth. They include the black stains caused by the products of tobacco combustion and the more or less characteristic *"metabolic"* stain thought to arise from chromogenic bacteria. Tobacco stains are dark brown or black and discolor the teeth diffusely in areas where there are adherent mucinous plaques present. Tobacco stains are present most often on the lingual surfaces of the teeth, especially in those areas where pipes, cigars, or cigarettes are held (Fig. 111). The degree of staining is generally related more to the degree of malhygiene than to the amount of smoking done. A black stain in the form of a fine line adjacent to the free gingival margin, which is not related to smoking, has been called metabolic stain and "mesenteric line." This stain may occur as a broad or thin black line following the contour of the free gingival margin onto the interproximal surfaces of the teeth (Fig. 112). It appears most frequently in women and in mouths receiving fastidious home care. It may be present on both the labial and lingual aspects of the teeth, but it most often occurs on the lingual surfaces of the maxillary molars and bicuspid teeth. The cause of this stain is unknown but is probably related to chromogenic bacteria. Such black stains may be removed with some difficulty by polishing agents but tend to

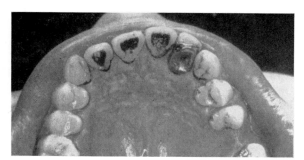

Figure 111. *Tobacco stain.* Heavy, black tar-like material deposited on protected areas of the maxillary teeth.

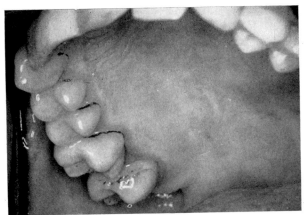

Figure 112. *Metabolic stain.* Deposit of a fine black line of stain on the palatal cervical area of the teeth.

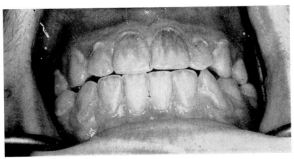

Figure 113. *Green stain.* Brownish-green, tenacious moss-like material on cervical one-third of labial surfaces of maxillary incisors.

recur promptly in many instances. Removal is sometimes more difficult because of pitting of the underlying enamel.

GREEN STAIN. A rather characteristic green stain frequently occurs on the teeth of children, especially on the cervical third of the labial surfaces of the maxillary incisors (Fig. 113). This stain may or may not be associated with the remains of the enamel cuticle. Not infrequently the enamel beneath this stain is roughened and predisposes to the formation of mucinous plaques and the recurrence of the stain. Roughened surfaces should be thoroughly polished to prevent the recurrence of the stain in soft mucinous plaques which form easily and adhere to rough surfaces.

ORANGE STAIN. Orange and red stains may be present on the teeth in various locations but more especially on the cervical third of the teeth. Such stains are related to soft plaques on the teeth and to the action of chromogenic bacteria. They are easily removed by polishing agents and may be effectively prevented by proper tooth-brushing.

Endogenous Stains

Internal discoloration of the teeth may occur as the result of decomposition of blood pigments associated with the death of the pulp. Such pigments give the tooth a grayish or blue-black discoloration (Fig. 114). The teeth occasionally may be discolored by blood-borne pigments associated with severe systemic diseases or inborn errors of pigment metabolism such as congenital porphyria. Endogenous stains may occur with the symptoms of severe jaundice due to systemic disease. The presence of an excess of bile pigments in the blood while the teeth are forming may discolor the teeth yellow or shades of yellow-green. In congenital porphyria the teeth are initially discolored various shades of red. A yellow to bluish-brown color can be produced in the teeth when tetracycline is incorporated in dentin and enamel during calcification. If tetracycline is administered to a pregnant woman during the time the fetus's teeth are forming or to the infant postnatally, those teeth being formed will be discolored.

A pink to black discoloration of the teeth may also result from internal resorption of the teeth. Where much of the internal portions of the teeth have been lost, the pink color of the pulp gives the tooth involved a pink coloration. Injury to the pulp and decomposition of blood pigments give the teeth with internal resorption a black color. Drugs introduced into the pulp chamber of a tooth

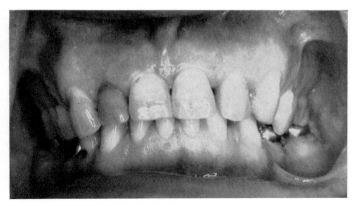

Figure 114. *Intrinsic stain.* Dark gray color of the entire crown of a lateral incisor is due to death of pulp.

may penetrate the dental tubules to cause discoloration of the tooth. In most instances the coloration is gray or black.

Discoloration of the teeth may also occur as the result of hereditary and developmental disturbances such as mottled enamel, amelogenesis imperfecta, dentinogenesis imperfecta, hereditary brown hypoplasia, and the use of tetracycline during pregnancy (Fig. 39). These discolorations are described in detail under developmental disturbances of the teeth.

SOFT ACCRETIONS

Various forms of soft accretions occur upon the teeth and are generally indicative of malhygiene. All areas of the mouth are subject to the deposition of soft accretions made up of varying amounts of mucin, bacteria, food debris, and epithelial cells. Soft organic accretions on the teeth include materia alba, mucinous and bacterial plaques, and the "pigmented pellicle."

MATERIA ALBA. Materia alba is a soft creamy white cheese-like substance occurring on the teeth of individuals exhibiting gross oral malhygiene. It most often occurs in the region of the gingival margin, but may cover the labial surfaces and lingual surfaces of the crown (Fig. 115). It is composed of food debris, mucin, dead cells, and various bacteria which are, at times, acid-forming. These accumulations are easily removed from the teeth by brushing and polishing. This type of accretion is seen most often on teeth out of occlusion or malposed, especially those which are not cleansed by natural factors and by home-care procedures. Mucinous films, bacterial plaques, and inorganic accretions are usually also present. Occasionally there is decalcification of the underlying enamel along the free gingival margins of the teeth. Such decalcified areas ap-

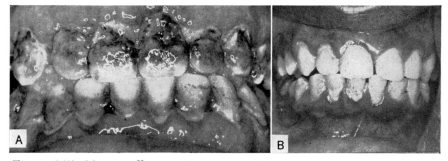

Figure 115. *Materia alba.* A, Heavy accumulation of soft and somewhat pigmented debris on surfaces of teeth which are not self-cleansing. This is an exaggerated situation. B, Accumulation of somewhat more solid type of materia alba along the gingival margin. This is the more usual appearance of materia alba than that on the left.

pear as white opaque linear and porous areas of enamel adjacent to the free border of the gingiva (Fig. 116). These decalcified areas are present more occlusally or incisally if gingival recession has occurred. Proteolytic organisms and their toxic products present in materia alba cause gingival irritation. This accretion must be differentiated from the pseudomembrane in Vincent's infection.

MUCINOUS PLAQUES. When the teeth are not brushed for a day or two, or where the brush has not reached certain areas, a white, somewhat transparent film called a dental plaque forms on the teeth. Such plaques may be easily removed by tooth-brushing but cannot be removed simply by rinsing with water. Dental plaques are readily demonstrated by the use of disclosing solution (Fig. 117), and, when the teeth are dried, the plaques present a non-

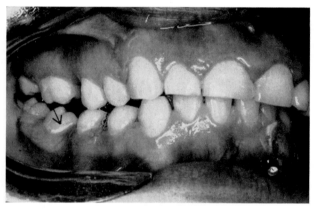

Figure 116. *Cervical decalcification.* Opaque line at cervical margin of malposed lower second molar. This area retained materia alba resulting in decalcification of the enamel. Materia alba can be seen on the other malposed molar teeth.

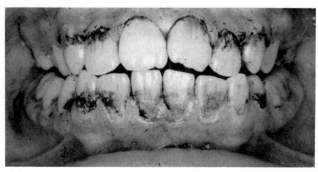

Figure 117. *Mucinous plaques* stained with disclosing solution are evident in areas that are not self-cleansing.

reflecting surface. Mucinous plaques may be discolored by pigmented foods, by chromogenic bacteria, and by metals or their salts. Plaques consist of mucin, food debris, bacteria, fungi, and epithelial cells. Although the formation of the plaque is not well understood, bacterial, chemical, and physical changes appear to be responsible. It is probable that microorganisms, especially of the filamentous type, become attached to the surface of the teeth to form a mesh or mat for the deposition of food and cellular debris. It is likely that the bacteria provide a properly acid media for the precipitation of mucin from the saliva. Alternate wetting and drying of this mucinous matrix might well enhance its solidification and attachment to the surface of the teeth. Dental plaques are significant in the formation of dental calculus, the production of dental caries, and the production of gingival irritation.

PIGMENTED PELLICLE. A noncellular brown keratin-like plaque that may be removed in strips occasionally is present on the teeth adjacent to the free gingival margins. This type of plaque is much more adherent than the mucinous plaque described above. The etiology of this pigmented pellicle is unknown, but it is thought to occur on the teeth of those individuals who brush their teeth regularly but use a nonabrasive dentifrice.

CALCULUS

Dental calculus is a hard accretion attached to surfaces of the teeth and principally consists of calcium phosphate arranged in an apatite lattice similar to bone and enamel. The structural arrangement is that of hydroxyapatite along with variable amounts of organic amorphous material. The inorganic constituents include calcium, phosphate, magnesium, and carbonates; the organic constituents include proteins (mucin, keratin, nucleoproteins), bacteria, cellular debris, and water. Chemical analysis has shown that approximately 80 percent of the inorganic constituents are calcium, magnesium, phosphate, and carbonate. Many filamentous microorganisms, such as leptotrichia and actinomyces, can be identified microscopically. Calculus occurs in all areas of the mouth from early adolescence to old age. These deposits are not often found on the teeth of children except in the presence of destructive periodontal disease. Calculus formation tends to increase with age. Calculus generally is classified according to its position on the tooth relative to the free gingival margin. Deposits located on the exposed surfaces of the teeth and coronally to the gingival crevice are designated supragingival calculus, whereas those located apically to the free gingival margin are designated subgingival calculus. The basic structure and composition of supragingival and subgingival calculus are the same.

SUPRAGINGIVAL CALCULUS. Calcifying or calcified masses of visible calcareous accretions may occur throughout the mouth on teeth not adequately cleansed by natural or artificial measures. The greatest quantity is usually present on those surfaces of the teeth opposite the openings of the ducts of the major salivary glands, i.e., the buccal surfaces of the maxillary molar teeth and the lingual surfaces of the mandibular anterior teeth (Fig. 118). If undisturbed, extremely large masses of calculus may form, even to the extent of covering the surfaces of the teeth and bridging the interproximal spaces or attaching to prosthetic appliances (Fig. 119). Such deposits are usually white or whitish-yellow but may be stained by pigments, tobacco, or other colored substances taken into the mouth (Fig. 120). The hardness of the calculus is dependent upon the degree of calcification. Supragingival calculus may be fairly easily

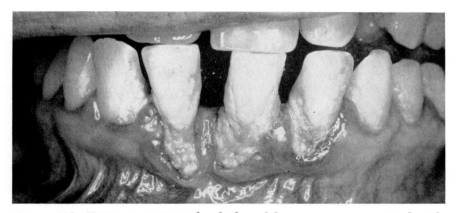

Figure 118. *Heavy supragingival calculus* of lower incisors associated with malposition and hypofunction of the teeth.

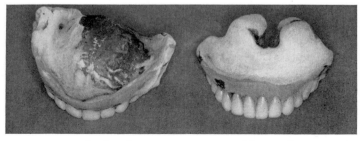

Figure 119. Heavy calculus deposits on upper and lower dentures which had not been removed from the mouth for several years.

detached with a scaler when calculus occurs only on the smooth surfaces of the enamel. However, in the presence of gingival recession where supragingival calculus is attached to the cementum and cemento-enamel junction, detachment may be considerably more difficult. The tenacity and hardness of these deposits are dependent on the smoothness of the enamel and cemental surfaces and on the degree of calcification.

SUBGINGIVAL CALCULUS. Calcular accretions located apically to the free gingival margin are best located by probing with an explorer, but well-calcified masses of calculus may also be seen radiographically (Fig. 121). Because of the assumption that the source of calcium in subgingival calculus was of blood serum origin, it was called "serumal calculus," but this assumption has not been substantiated. Subgingival deposits of calculus involving the cementum

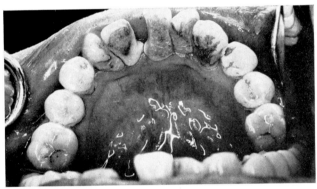

Figure 120. *Supragingival deposits of calculus on lower incisor.* This is the most frequent location of calculus. The color is that seen in smokers. Note the bridging effect produced by the heavy deposits.

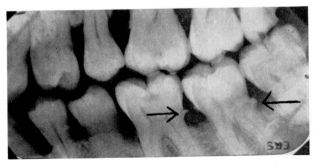

Figure 121. Radiograph demonstrating spurs of subgingival calculus on mandibular first and second molars.

are firmly attached and are more difficult to remove than calcareous deposits occurring on the enamel surfaces. Subgingival deposits may occur in plate-like accretions, granular deposits, ledges, or nodular masses. These deposits may extend from the base of the gingival crevice or periodontal pocket to the free gingival margin and may extend coronally to blend in with supragingival deposits. Such deposits may occur with or without the presence of significant amounts of supragingival calculus. Subgingival deposits may be white, grayish, brown, black, or greenish-black in color. The hardness of calculus and the tenacity of its attachment are generally proportional to the degree of calcification and to the roughness of the surfaces to which it is attached, but vary considerably from one individual to another.

Formation of Calculus

A variety of factors appears to be related to the formation of dental calculus. The exact mechanism by which calculus is formed has not been clearly established on the basis of either clinical observation or laboratory investigation. Most of the theories regarding the mechanism of calculus formation are based on physical, chemical, or bacterial conditions in the mouth. Theories related to systemic (body) disturbances have also been suggested but have gained little acceptance. Most of the physicochemical theories are related to factors which might facilitate the precipitation of calcium salts from the saliva. Thus, many factors which would tend to decrease the solubility of calcium salts in the saliva have been suggested as responsible for the formation of calculus.

Saliva is normally a saturated solution of calcium phosphate with respect to the blood and enamel. The concentration of calcium phosphate ions in solution in saliva is a reflection of the solubility of calcium phosphate and the pH of the saliva. The pH of the saliva varies from individual to individual and in the same individual throughout the day. The average pH of the saliva is just below neutral or pH 7. A pH below 7 is on the acid side of neutral, whereas a pH above 7 is on the alkaline side. Ordinarily the saliva is buffered by phosphates, carbonates, and proteins to resist any change in the hydrogen ion concentration. Factors that tend to keep the inorganic salts in solution in the saliva include hydrogen ions (acids), proteins, and carbon dioxide. Factors that tend to facilitate the precipitation of inorganic salts from the saliva are hydroxyl ions (bases), loss of salivary proteins, and loss of carbon dioxide. When the pH of the saliva is changed, its ability to hold calcium and phosphate ions in solution is altered accordingly. When carbon dioxide is lost from the saliva, the pH of the saliva is shifted to the alkaline side, which is a factor in reducing the solubility of calcium phosphate and its precipitation as calculus. Although the buffering system previously mentioned generally protects the saliva from such a change, localized areas such as those opposite the salivary gland ducts may be sufficiently alkaline for short periods of time to favor the precipitation of inorganic salts. The loss of carbon dioxide also favors the loss of calcium phosphate from solution in the saliva, inasmuch as carbon dioxide itself apparently favors the maintenance of calcium in solution by the formation of a complex ion with calcium. The carbon dioxide loss theory for the formation of calculus appears to account for the tendency of calculus to form readily on those teeth nearest the salivary ducts, since large amounts of carbon dioxide might be expected to be lost from the saliva as it comes from the ducts of the salivary glands.

Bacterial theories of calculus formation suggest that bacteria directly or indirectly enter into the formation of calculus by forming an organic framework for the deposition of calcium salts, by producing centers of alkalinity, or by producing enzymes which act as trigger mechanisms in the precipitation of calcium salts. There is no unanimity of opinion about the role that bacteria play in regard to bacterial decomposition of protein and liberation of organic-bound calcium in the saliva, since the amount liberated would be too small to be significant. For the same reason most investigators feel that the enzyme, phosphatase, derived from bacteria is not a significant factor in the relase of organic phosphates from the saliva. It is probable that changes in the plaque as well as the saliva occur at intervals and in short periods of time. That calculus formation is intermittent is based on microscopic examination of specimens of calculus which show a laminated structure.

The attachment of calculus to the teeth appears to be dependent upon the presence of filamentous organisms and the irregularity of the tooth surface (Fig. 122). Rough surfaces of the enamel and cementum favor the penetration of filamentous microorganisms making up the organic matrix of the plaque and, thus, make possible a mechanical bond between the tooth structure and the calcifying plaque. Therefore, it is imperative that all tooth surfaces be as smooth as possible to inhibit the attachment of the organic matrix which predisposes to the formation of calculus. It is also imperative that home-care procedures are directed toward the removal of plaques before their calcification begins in 12 to 15 hours or less. From the foregoing discussion it is obvious that oral hygiene can influence the amount of calculus formed; however, it does not appear to be related to the actual mechanism of calculus formation. This is also true of the ammonia produced by bacteria. Thus, the

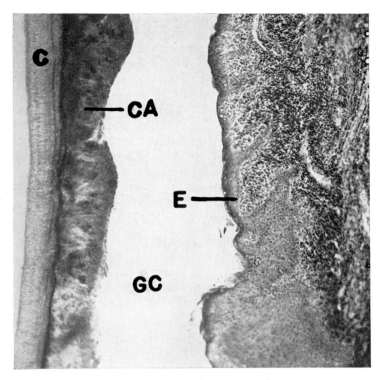

Figure 122. *Attachment of subgingival deposit of calculus to cementum.* Note inflammation of the adjacent gingiva. Cementum, (C); calculus, (CA); crevicular epithelium, (E); pathologically deepened gingival crevice, (GC).

most widely accepted bacterial theory at the present time is related to the formation of a mat or organic framework for the deposition of calcium salts. The factors within this organic mat that favor the precipitation of inorganic salts is not clear.

Although the exact mechanism for the formation of calculus is not known, it may well occur in the following manner: initially, a plaque of soft material composed of mucin, epithelial debris, and bacteria forms on an area of tooth surface not cleaned by normal action of saliva, tongue, lips, cheeks, or by the action of a toothbrush. Thus, the stage preceding calculus formation consists of the attachment of a bacterial or mucinous plaque to the surface of the teeth. After the plaque has begun to form, it presents an organic matrix for the deposition of inorganic salts. If the plaque is undisturbed, physical, chemical, and bacterial changes occur locally in the plaque which are favorable to the precipitation and calcification of the plaque. Calcification of the plaque begins in a relatively short period of time. While the exact factors responsible for the precipitation of calcium salts in the plaque are not established, it appears that the loss of carbon dioxide from the saliva is capable of shifting the pH of saliva locally to the extent that is becomes supersaturated with calcium salts to the point of precipitation even in the presence of scrupulous oral hygiene, and calculus formation occurs at a rapid rate. This fact does not lessen the practical importance of removing plaques, since their quick removal diminishes the amount of calculus which will be formed; however, it does point out that the inherent tendency of some individuals to form calculus more rapidly than others is not simply a matter of poor oral hygiene or the mechanical removal of plaques, but some factor intimately related to the mechanism of the formation of calculus.

BIBLIOGRAPHY

Bevelander, G., Hiroshi, N., and Rolbe, G. H.: The effect of the administration of tetracycline on the development of teeth. J. Dent. Res., 40:1020, 1961.
Bibby, B. G.: The formation of salivary calculus. Dent. Cosmos, 77:668, 1935.
Bulleid, A.: A symposium on calculus. The bacteriologic aspect. Dent. Pract., 4:224, 1954.
Gregg, J. M.: The tetracycline antibiotics: A dental challenge in 1964. Univ. of Mich. Alumni Bull., Oct. 1964.
Hodge, H. C., and Leung, S. W.: Calculus formation. J. Periodont., 21:211, 1950.
Leung, S. W., and Jensen, A. T.: Factors controlling deposition of calculus. Int. Dent. J., 8:613, 1958.
Mello, H. S.: The mechanism of tetracycline staining in primary and permanent teeth. J. Dent. Child., 34:478, 1967.
Prinz, H.: The origin of salivary calculus. Dent. Cosmos, 63:231, 1921.
Rapp, G. W.: Biochemistry of oral calculus; I. Conditions predisposing to oral calculus deposition. J. Amer. Dent. Ass., 32:1368, 1945.
Weyman, J., and Porteus, J. R.: Discoloration of teeth possibly due to administration of tetracycline. Brit. Dent. J., 11:351, 1962.
Zander, H. A.: Attachment of calculus to root surfaces. J. Periodont., 24:16, 1953.

Chapter 11

PERIODONTAL DISEASE

Periodontal disease refers to disturbances which are unique to the periodontium because of its form and function. Thus, the term refers to diseases which occur primarily because of, but not incidental to, the presence of the periodontal structures. In this sense, gingivitis and periodontitis are examples of periodontal disease, whereas other types of lesions, such as oral manifestations of dermatologic disorders involving the periodontium, are not unique to the periodontium and cannot be considered as periodontal disease, viz., herpetic gingivostomatitis. Basically, the pathologic processes found elsewhere in the body, such as inflammation and progressive and retrogressive changes, also involve the periodontium. However, since the periodontium comprises rather unique structures, pathologic processes give rise to rather special anatomic, histologic, and functional changes which require special terminology, evaluation, and treatment. In order to facilitate an understanding of periodontal disease, a brief review of the normal histologic and clinical features of the periodontium follows.

PERIODONTIUM

The periodontium consists of the investing and supporting structures of the teeth and includes the periodontal membrane, the gingiva, the alveolar bone, and the cementum. These structures are arranged as a functional unit primarily for the support of the teeth. The interdependence of these structures both anatomically and physiologically is a reflection of their origin, development, and maintenance. The cementum is considered part of the periodontium because, like the alveolar bone, it is a product of the mesenchymal tissue of the periodontal membrane and periodontal fibers are inserted into it.

PERIODONTAL MEMBRANE. The periodontal membrane is the specialized connective tissue surrounding the roots of the teeth and is responsible for the support of the teeth. It also is responsible for the formation and nutrition of the alveolar bone, cementum, and

15

principal fibers, and for sensory perception of pressure, tension, heat, cold, and pain. Much of the connective tissue of the periodontal membrane is arranged into bundles or groups of fibers to counteract any force applied to the tooth from any direction. The parts of the principal fibers which are inserted into the cementum and bone are called Sharpey's fibers. Interspersed between the bundles of principal fibers are the nerves and vessels supplying the periodontal membrane. The principal fibers are oriented so that forces applied to the tooth are transmitted to the alveolar bone as tension. This tension, mediated through the principal fibers and their attachment to the bone, is conducive to the formation and maintenance of bone. The periodontal membrane varies in width depending upon the degree of function to which the tooth is exposed, the age of the individual, and the area of the root involved. The width of the periodontal membrane is greater when there is hyperfunction of the teeth than when there is hypofunction. The width is also greater at the cervical and apical regions of the teeth than in the fulcrum areas of the roots of the teeth. The periodontal membrane as well as the cementum and alveolar bone is continually undergoing changes to meet the functional demands of the teeth. Physiologic and pathologic changes involving eruption and movement of the teeth require the principal fibers to be continually reformed and reoriented and reattached to the alveolar bone and cementum.

ALVEOLAR BONE. The alveolar bone (alveolar bone proper) is that bone which is continuous with the lateral cortical plates of the alveolar process and which is adjacent to the periodontal membrane. It forms the walls of the sockets of the teeth into which the principal fibers of the periodontal membrane are attached. The *alveolar process* is the portion of the mandible and maxilla forming the jaw and supporting the alveolar bone and teeth. It consists of cancellous bone surrounded by dense cortical plate. Radiographically, it is a finger-like projection of cancellous bone seen between the teeth and supports the alveolar bone proper and the alveolar crest (Fig. 123).

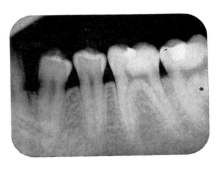

Figure 123. *Normal alveolar bone and lamina dura.* Note fine white line extending around root and over bone crest between teeth.

The alveolar crest is seen radiographically as a continuation of the alveolar bone proper over the crest of the alveolar process. Anatomically, it is the interproximal or interdental rim of the alveolar socket. The term *lamina dura* is used to describe the radiographic appearance of the alveolar bone proper. As in other areas of the body, the alveolar bone is highly plastic tissue and has the characteristic of adaptation to functional stimuli. The maintenance and replacement of alveolar bone represent a state of equilibrium between resorption and formation. Thus, bone is constantly resorbed and reformed to meet functional stimuli; this process becomes more highly active in the presence of movement of teeth, injury of teeth, and extraction of teeth. In the absence of teeth and functional stimuli, the alveolar process tends to be resorbed. During orthodontic movement of the teeth, the alveolar bone is resorbed and reformed to meet the requirements of the new positions of the teeth. In the presence of injury, the process of bone resorption may be more active than bone formation. As previously mentioned, tension to bone mediated through the principal fibers is conducive to the formation of bone, whereas pressure is conducive to its resorption (Fig. 124–1, 2). Thus, if a force is directed on a tooth in a

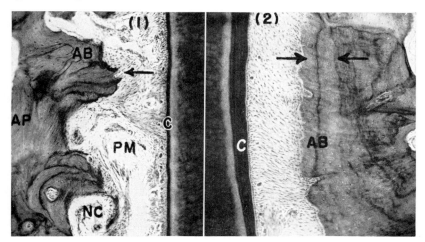

Figure 124. *Periodontal changes with movement of teeth.* Photomicrographs showing mesial movement of a tooth. 1, Mesial surface (side of pressure) of alveolar bone. AB shows resorption of alveolar bone. Arrow indicates Howship's lacunae where bone is being resorbed. Periodontal membrane, PM; alveolar process, AP; nutrient canal, NC; cementum C. Note small round structures below C adjacent to cementum—these are epithelial rests. 2, Distal surface (side of tension) of alveolar bone. Note fine dark line between arrows—this is a growth line between two zones of bone formed in response to tension.

mesial direction, resorption and formation of bone are to be expected in the sites of pressure and tension. In this instance, the site of resorption will be on the mesial aspect of the root and formation of bone on the distal aspect of the root. When the force is removed, for example when an orthodontic appliance is removed, the ordinary rate of resorption and reformation of bone necessary for the maintenance of the tooth in its position will again take place.

A radiographic examination of the alveolar bone proper and the alveolar process under normal conditions shows that the lamina dura (alveolar bone proper) is continuous throughout the mouth. A lack of continuity is indicative of a disease process. A lack of continuity of the lamina dura is seen most frequently in the region of the alveolar crest and apices of the teeth. The former is generally related to periodontal disease and the latter to disease of the pulp. The height of the alveolar crest should be within 1 to 1½ millimeters of the cemento-enamel junction (Fig. 123). The form of the alveolar crest between the teeth is related to the position of the adjacent teeth and to the shape of the teeth.

CEMENTUM. Cementum is continuously deposited throughout the life of the teeth. The continuous deposition is necessary for reattachment of the principal fibers loosened by movement of the teeth and to repair injury. Cementum is not resorbed under normal conditions except in association with the resorption of the roots of the primary dentition. Because of the continued deposition of cementum and the formation of alveolar bone, the width of the periodontal membrane remains relatively uniform. The fact that cementum is less likely to resorb than bone makes orthodontic movement of the teeth possible.

The relationship of the cementum to the enamel shows considerable variation. In most instances, the cementum will slightly overlap the enamel to form the cemento-enamel junction. Less frequently, there is an edge-to-edge approximation of the cementum and enamel; even less frequently, the cementum and enamel fail to meet. In the first instance, cementum overlapping the enamel may be mistaken for a ridge of calculus during scaling. The approximation of the cementum to the enamel is of considerable importance in periodontal disease and in root scaling.

Occlusal forces on the teeth may influence the amount and location of the deposition of cementum. Hypercementosis, cemental spikes, and cemental tears may be associated with traumatic occlusion. Resorption of the cementum and of the roots may occur from excessive function and orthodontic movement of the teeth. Rough and/or soft cementum is conducive to the attachment of dental plaques and calculus and thus to the initiation and progression of periodontal disease.

GINGIVA. The gingiva is a specialized portion of the mucous membranes of the mouth which surround the cervical region of the teeth and cover the alveolar processes. The gingiva is divided clinically and histologically into the free gingiva, the attached gingiva, and the interdental papilla. The *free gingiva* is the "unattached" gingiva surrounding the teeth and forming the wall of the gingival crevice. The *attached gingiva* is the part of the gingiva attached to the underlying cementum and the alveolar bone. It extends from the free gingival margin to the oral mucosa. The attached gingiva is supported by a dense, firm connective tissue that fuses with the periosteum of the alveolar process. The *interdental papilla* is the portion of the gingiva which fills the interproximal space.

The clinical evaluation of the gingiva is based upon its color, form, density, and attachment. Normal gingiva is uniformly pale pink in color. Physiologic pigmentation also may be present to alter its color uniformity and shade (Fig. 125). The pigmentation of the gingiva is generally related to an individual's skin pigmentation. The color of the gingiva is dependent upon its vascularity, keratinization, and the presence or absence of inflammation. In acute inflammation, the pale-pink color is altered to varying shades of red. In areas of chronic inflammation, the color is generally altered to

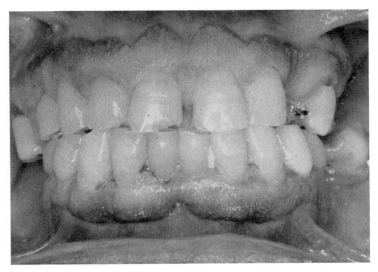

Figure 125. *Pigmentation and stippling.* Dark areas of the attached gingiva are areas of melanin pigment of the type seen in dark-skinned people. Stippling is slightly more prominent than normal.

show a bluish shade (cyanosis). Thus, the normal color of the gingiva is altered because of the presence of passive congestion where an absolute increase in the amount of reduced hemoglobin of the blood occurs (5 gm/100 cc).

The form of the gingiva is related to the form of the crowns of the teeth, the spacing of the teeth, the form of the alveolar processes, the contour of the roots of the teeth, and to the presence of disease. In a normal mouth the gingiva fills the interproximal spaces and is closely adapted to the surfaces of the teeth (Fig. 126). In the presence of periodontal disease, the normal form of the gingiva is lost

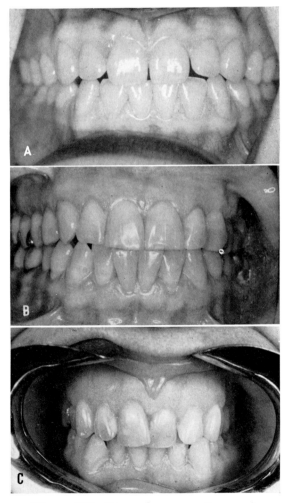

Figure 126. (*Legend on opposite page.*)

so that the free gingival margin is no longer closely adapted to the surfaces of the teeth, and the interdental papillae are enlarged and overfill the interproximal spaces (Fig. 140). The interdental papilla also may be lost leaving open embrasures between the teeth.

The density of the normal gingiva is firm and resilient to palpation. The presence of periodontal disease alters the normal density of the gingiva and gives the gingiva a soft, spongy character. Stippling of the gingiva analogous to the skin of an orange is present in the absence of disease. In some instances when gingival crevices are pathologically deepened, stippling may be present where active chronic inflammation is limited to the base of the gingival crevice or periodontal pocket.

The *epithelial attachment* is the portion of the gingiva attached to the surfaces of the teeth. The epithelial attachment of the gingiva of a normal young adult should be on the enamel or at the cemento-enamel junction. It moves apically with advancing age, and, in late adult life, it is on the cementum with about a millimeter of the cementum exposed. The presence of the epithelial attachment on

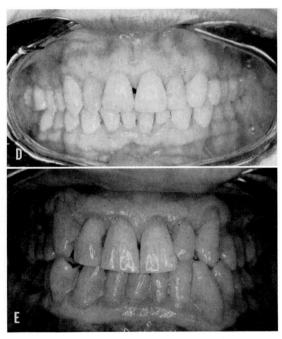

Figure 126. *Normal gingiva.* Gingival tissue showing the physiologic recession (eruption) at various years of age: A, 20 years; B, 52 years; C, 60 years; D, 71 years; E, 80 years. All are considered normal for the stated ages.

the cementum of a young individual should be considered pathologic and the result of disease, but would be considered physiologic for a person of advanced age. When there is simultaneous atrophy of the alveolar crest and gingiva and apical migration of the epithelial attachment beyond the cemento-enamel junction, physiologic recession has taken place.

The *gingival crevice* or gingival sulcus is the shallow groove which develops between the gingiva and the surfaces of the tooth. It is formed by the boundaries of the gingiva and the surfaces of the teeth. The normal depth of the gingival crevice in an adult does not exceed 2 to 3 millimeters. The base of the gingival crevice or sulcus is the epithelial attachment. An increase in the depth of the gingival crevice occurs as the result of periodontal disease. An increase in the depth of the gingival crevice may occur as the result of hyperplasia of the gingiva and/or apical migration of the epithelial attachment, as in a periodontal pocket. A periodontal pocket is a pathologic deepening of the gingival crevice associated with the loss of supporting structures and apical migration of the epithelial attachment. A deepening of the gingival crevice involving only hyperplasia of the gingiva, and not apical migration of the epithelial attachment beyond the cemento-enamel junction, is regarded as a "relative" pocket and not a true periodontal pocket. Such pockets are designated as pseudo- or gingival pockets.

In order to appreciate the goals of periodontal therapy and the maintenance of oral hygiene, the criteria for a *healthy gingiva* as well as a normal gingiva should also be considered. The criteria for a normal gingiva are useful in determining the presence and extent of periodontal disease; the criteria of a healthy gingiva are useful in evaluating the form and attachment of the gingiva after the normal form and attachment have been altered. A normal gingiva is a healthy one; however, a healthy gingiva may not have normal form and attachment. The color of a healthy gingiva is uniformly pale pink, except as altered by physiologic pigmentation. The form of the gingiva may be altered and no longer fill the interproximal spaces to the contact area. Even so, the free gingival margin should be closely adapted to the surfaces of the teeth if it is to remain healthy. For example, in gingival recession or following the loss of interdental papilla by necrotizing gingivitis or gingivectomy, the important consideration is that the depth of the crevice be no greater than 3 millimeters and that the free gingival margin be closely adapted to the surfaces of the teeth. The gingiva is considered as healthy if the foregoing criteria of a healthy gingiva are met even though the epithelial attachment is on the cementum. Thus, the position of the epithelial attachment in a healthy gingiva is irrelevant provided the color, form, and density of the gingiva, and the depth of the gingival crevice are functionally healthy.

EPIDEMIOLOGY

Epidemiology is the study of the mass phenomenon of disease and is not necessarily limited to contagious diseases. Epidemiologic studies have been undertaken to determine the susceptibility of different racial, geographic, cultural, economic, and ethnic groups to periodontal disease. Such studies have been undertaken to determine the effectiveness of therapeutic measures in the control and prevention of dental and periodontal diseases, viz., fluoride in drinking water, periodic prophylaxis, and tooth-brushing. Epidemiologic studies have considered the importance of various etiologic factors in the production of periodontal disease, viz., the role of smoking in the etiology of gingivitis. The results of epidemiologic studies often are reported in terms of incidence or prevalence of a disease. The *incidence* of disease refers to the number of cases of a disease that occurs in a given period of time per unit of population, viz., 50 cases of measles occurred for every 10,000 children in one year (rate). *Prevalence* refers to the number of cases of a disease found at a particular time in a unit of population, viz., one case of cleft palate is found in every 1000 individuals. Incidence usually refers to contagious disease, accidents, or deaths; prevalence refers to congenital disease, developmental diseases, and diseases of insidious onset with vague or no termination. Thus, one may speak of the incidence of Vincent's infection and the prevalence of periodontitis. The information derived from epidemiologic studies has been useful in determining the nature and etiology of periodontal disease and has provided sufficient evidence to strongly support the view that periodontal disease constitutes a serious public health problem.

The results of epidemiologic studies indicate that the prevalence and severity of gingival disease generally increase with age. Gingivitis in children rises sharply with the eruption of the permanent teeth from six to eight years of age and continues to the age of puberty, following which it falls sharply until the late teens. After the early twenties the prevalence and severity of gingival disease steadily increase to the age of 50 and above when the prevalence of gingivitis reaches almost 100 percent. It is apparent from epidemiologic studies that the prevalence of gingival disease in children and in adolescents reaches approximately 75 percent. It is apparent that the end of puberty and the final eruption of the teeth are in part responsible for the downward trend in the prevalence of gingivitis during late adolescence. Probably a greater emphasis on oral hygiene and esthetics at the end of puberty and during late adolescence are factors in the decreasing prevalence of gingivitis at this age. It has been found that girls demonstrate better oral hygiene during the late teens than boys. Thus sex differences appear to be quite important in the late teens and early twenties, since 75 percent of the boys show gingival disease compared to approximately 50 percent of the girls. This sex difference in the prevalence of gingival disease becomes less evident with the development of chronic destructive periodontal disease.

Chronic destructive periodontal disease, which involves a loss of the alveolar bone, appears to be relatively low in young children but increases rather slowly and continuously up to 20 years of age. After this age the prevalence of chronic destructive periodontal disease with bone loss increases rapidly from about 24 percent at the age of 19 to 69 percent at the age of 26. By the age of 45 epidemiologic studies indicate the prevalence of chronic destructive periodontal disease to be almost 100 percent. By the age of 35 more teeth are lost from periodontal disease than from all other causes. Despite the high tooth mortality due to periodontal disease, only a relatively small percentage of affected individuals are aware of the presence of periodontal disease, and even a smaller number have received any treatment. These findings indicate that the prevention or treatment of periodontal disease early in life could lead to a significant reduction in the loss of teeth due to periodontal disease. Furthermore, there is sufficient reliable epidemiologic evidence to support the view that poor oral hygiene is a significant factor in the production of periodontal disease.

ETIOLOGY

The etiologic factors or causes of periodontal disease may be divided, for discussion purposes, into two groups: (1) initiating or local factors which cause injury to the periodontium, and (2) modifying or contributory factors which influence the reaction of the tissues to injury. Obviously such a division is arbitrary, and all periodontal disease can be considered to be the result of both initiating and modifying factors. Even so, this division of etiologic factors is basic to an understanding of the cause of periodontal disease. Such a grouping of etiologic factors proposes that all periodontal disease (as previously defined) is primarily a reaction of the periodontal tissues to injury. Thus from a practical standpoint, in the treatment and prevention of periodontal disease, the factors initiating the injury constitute the most important group of causative factors of periodontal disease. This "reaction-to-injury" concept of the etiology of periodontal disease leads to the forthright inference that periodontal disease can be prevented by eliminating the local and surface irritants which injure periodontal tissues. The reaction of the periodontal tissues to injury is manifested as gingivitis and periodontitis. The severity of the reaction to local irritation is dependent upon the magnitude of the local factors and the modification of the tissue response by systemic factors. The following is a summary of the initiating and modifying factors responsible for periodontal disease.

A. *Initiating Factors*

    1. Surface irritants
        Calculus, materia alba, dental plaques, bacteria
    2. Faulty dentistry
        Overhanging margins of restorations, open contacts, improper marginal ridges, porous filling materials, lack of functional contours
    3. Mouth-breathing

B. *Modifying (Contributory) Factors*

    1. Dysfunctional factors
        Malposed teeth, unilateral mastication, traumatic occlusion, loss of teeth
    2. Systemic factors
        Hormonal imbalance, nutritional deficiencies, metabolic errors, resistance, constitution, hereditary factors.

Initiating Factors

The initiation of periodontal disease primarily involves poor oral hygiene because of the presence of materia alba, dental plaques, and calculus, which produce chemical, bacterial, and mechanical irritation of the periodontium. There can be no doubt that surface irritants, such as calculus and dental plaques, are primarily responsible for the initiation of periodontal disease, since these irritants are always present in periodontal disease. It is significant that the inflammatory response subsides with the removal of the local irritants and the establishment of good oral hygiene. The degree of inflammatory response or severity of periodontal disease is dependent in part upon the local factors which are present and in part upon the individual's local and general resistance to disease. A severe response to surface irritants may occur even when the irritant is difficult to detect clinically. Thus, a slight degree of irritation may initiate a severe inflammatory response in the periodontium because of contributory systemic factors. In other instances, large

amounts of surface irritants may produce only a minimal inflammatory response, probably because of the high local and systemic resistance of the individual.

SURFACE IRRITANTS. Dental plaques, materia alba (Fig. 115),
and calculus (Figs. 118, 121) are irritants of local origin which injure the gingiva. Calculus may produce injury to the gingiva (especially the unkeratinized crevicular epithelium) because of mechanical trauma from the hard, rough surfaces of the calculus. During
movement of the teeth and when pressure is placed on the gingiva,
the calculus produces physical injury to the soft tissues. The irritation of the gingiva, especially the gingival crevice, by plaques and
calculus leads to ulceration of the crevicular epithelium. Changes
in the local resistance of the tissues associated with inflammatory
response may result from interference of the blood supply, relative
anoxia, and trauma. Such changes and ulceration of the epithelium
predispose the tissues to the effects of microorganisms. The action
of microorganisms is not by direct invasion of healthy tissues, but
by the production of substances which facilitate the spread of
organisms and inflammation. These substances (enzymes) include
hyaluronidase, which acts to break down hyaluronic acid (an important component of connective tissue). Thus, bacterial toxins and
enzymes are important agents in the production and spread of
inflammation. The spread of gingivitis is an important consideration in the loss of the supporting structures of the teeth.

The removal of dental plaque, materia alba, and calculus is a
primary consideration in the prevention of periodontal disease. A
periodic prophylaxis and maintenance of good oral hygiene by the
patient are absolutely necessary to prevent the formation of dental
plaques, materia alba, and calculus and to prevent periodontal
disease.

Faulty dental restorations, manifested by overhanging margins,
faulty marginal ridges, and improper proximal contacts, are important factors in the causation of periodontal disease (Fig. 127). Poorly

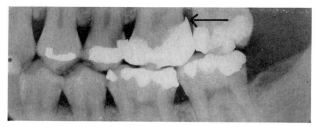

Figure 127. Local irritation produced by over-extended restoration indicated
by arrow. Note recurrent caries on the distal surface of the second
bicuspid.

constructed restorations or appliances often lead to mechanical injury of the tissues and the retention of food debris and bacteria. Food impaction may be the result of open proximal contact, faulty marginal ridges, and inadequate functional contouring of the restored surfaces of the teeth. Food wedged in the gingival crevice and in the interproximal areas leads to mechanical, chemical, and bacterial irritation. Food wedged in the teeth may also produce circulatory disturbances. If the impacted food is not removed, it will break down and ferment producing toxins and bacterial enzymes. The removal of overhanging margins of restorations and the prevention of food impaction are important duties of periodontal therapy. Ideally, dental restorations should be properly contoured and adapted to the teeth. The significance of proper contouring and of marginal adaptation of restorations in the production of periodontal disease is often overlooked. Porous filling materials, especially poorly processed acrylic and silicates, are detrimental to the soft tissues since they become impregnated with soft debris and bacteria and provide a basis for the attachment of plaques and calculus.

Faulty tooth-brushing and improper massage of the gingiva cause soft tissue laceration, pressure atrophy, and circulatory disturbances of the gingiva. Gingival recession frequently is present in association with cross-stroke or scrub-brush methods of brushing and where excessive pressure is applied (Fig. 128).

Mouth-breathing, which causes constant drying of the gingiva,

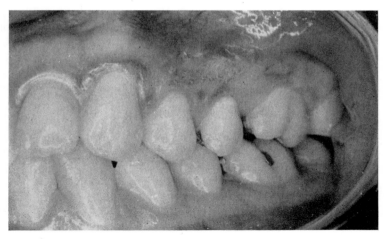

Figure 128. *Toothbrush injury.* Erosion and superficial ulceration of gingiva above bicuspid and first molar due to injury from improper toothbrushing.

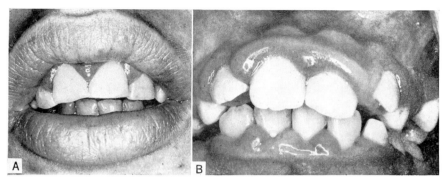

Figure 129. A, *Mouth-breather*. Note area of hyperplasia of interdental papillae not covered by the upper lip. B, *Mouth-breather*. Ridge-like hyperplasia of anterior gingiva ("tension ridge") due to increase in bulk of gingiva and pressure of lip.

produces gingival irritation (Fig. 129). Mouth-breathing may be a residual habit formed during childhood in response to tongue and lip habits associated with enlarged tonsils and adenoids. Mouth-breathing also may be related to the functional or organic obstruction of nasal passages. Functional obstruction may occur as the result of an enlarged venous bed in the nasal mucous membrane or allergic rhinitis. Organic nasal obstruction may be due to a deviated nasal septum, traumatic injury, or growths in the nasal passages. Gingival irritation associated with mouth-breathing is often rather sharply limited to the area of the gingiva left uncovered by the lips. Constant drying of the mucosa may be present in non-mouth-breathers when malposed and protruding teeth prevent normal closure of the lips.

Chemical, thermal, and mechanical irritants producing injury elsewhere in the mouth may cause gingival irritation. The use of tobacco in any form acts as an irritant. The mechanism by which this occurs may be related to heat, stains, deposits, or by-products of the tobacco. Caustic drugs, aspirin, toothache drops, and other medicaments are capable of producing an acute gingival inflammation. Such forms of irritation are discussed under stomatitis in Chapter 12, page 245.

Modifying (Contributory) Factors

Several factors contribute to the initiation and maintenance of periodontal disease and modify the response of the tissue to injury. Such contributory or modifying factors may be grouped into dysfunctional and systemic factors. Dysfunctional factors include hyperfunction and hypofunction of the teeth. Systemic factors include endocrine and nutritional disturbances and an individual's non-specific constitutional and resistive attributes which influence the response of the tissue to injury.

DYSFUNCTIONAL FACTORS. Dysfunctional irritation of the periodontium may result from traumatic occlusion arising from purposeless tapping, grinding, and gnashing of teeth (bruxism), loss of teeth, malpositioned teeth, and "high" restorations. Traumatic occlusion results in circulatory disturbances which interfere with the normal metabolic and functional characteristics of the periodontium. It may also cause hyperemia, inflammatory edema, degeneration, atrophy, and, in some instances, necrosis of the tissues of the periodontium. Minor injury associated with traumatic occlusion has an irritational effect on the vessels and cells of the periodontium and eventually leads to inflammation with exudation. Aside from the subtle changes of the tissues arising from minor injury of traumatic occlusion, disruption of the blood vessels, thrombosis and ischemic necrosis occur from severe trauma. Circulatory and metabolic disturbances are of special significance in the gingiva when the surface irritants, such as materia alba, dental plaque, and calculus, are present. Lowering the resistance of the periodontal tissues by traumatic occlusion predisposes to the extension of the inflammation, arising from surface irritants, into the supporting structures. Dysfunctional irritation arising from traumatic occlusion may also lead to periodontal atrophy and gingival recession. Occlusal dysfunction may bring about drifting and repositioning of teeth. It is not uncommon for patients who complain of the development of spaces between the teeth, especially anterior teeth, and of extrusion of teeth to exhibit occlusal imbalance and occlusal trauma (traumatism) (Fig. 130).

Hypofunction of the teeth occurs from nonocclusion, unilateral

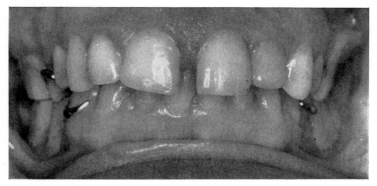

Figure 130. *Drifting of teeth* due to pressure produced by deep overbite and loss of posterior vertical dimension.

mastication, and tooth malposition. Teeth that are out of physiologic function or occlusion do not properly stimulate the supporting structures leading to disuse atrophy of the periodontal structures. Thus, hypofunction of the teeth leads to a lowering of the resistance of the supporting structures of the teeth. Even of greater significance is the fact that materia alba, dental plaque, and calculus tend to accumulate on teeth which are not actively used in mastication. This fact may be readily appreciated by observing the accumulation of plaque and calculus present on teeth which do not have an occluding tooth in the opposing arch. This same effect may also be noted in unilateral mastication. The side not used in mastication tends to accumulate soft debris and plaque and exhibits more gingivitis than the side used habitually.

SYSTEMIC FACTORS. Systemic disease per se does not produce periodontal disease. However, the response of the periodontium to local injuries which initiate the disease is reflected in the nutritional, hormonal, and metabolic state of the individual. In the absence of an injurious agent, no response of the tissues, as manifested by gingivitis or periodontitis, is to be anticipated. However, from a practical standpoint some degree of irritation exists in all mouths. The type and severity of the response to injury are dependent upon the local factors present and upon systemic influences which modify the response of the tissues to injury. In most instances, systemic influences on the periodontium cannot be altered and the treatment of periodontal disease is directed toward the removal of all the local factors initiating and contributing to the disease. Thus, rational periodontal therapy is directed toward the removal of local and dysfunctional irritants.

While adequate nutrition is an essential factor in the maintenance of a normal periodontium, there is little conclusive evidence to indicate that human nutritional deficiences are widespread or important specifically in the production of periodontal disease. So-called subclinical deficiencies of various vitamins, minerals, and other foodstuffs do not appear at this time to be clinically important in the production of periodontal disease, especially in view of the fact that periodontal disease can be adequately treated by the removal of surface and dysfunctional irritants. Vitamin C deficiency, especially subclinical deficiency of vitamin C, is often pointed out as the cause of gingivitis. In reality, however, even individuals with frank scurvy have little tendency to develop gingivitis in the absence of local and dysfunctional irritants (see p. 161).

Hormonal imbalance is potentially capable of modifying the response of the gingiva to irritation. The fact that rather severe responses of the gingiva to irritation may occur in puberty and in pregnancy has been attributed to hormonal imbalance during these altered physiologic states. In puberty and pregnancy the usual response of the tissues to injury is exaggerated so that varying degrees of gingival hyperplasia or enlargement may be seen. Histologically, the inflammatory response is not specific in character and cannot be attributed to pregnancy or puberty unless the physical state of the patient is known.

Pregnancy gingivitis is not a specific form of gingivitis but rather a nonspecific exaggerated response of the gingiva to surface irritants. Such a response is manifested near the end of the first trimester of pregnancy. Clinically, the systemic influence of pregnancy appears to cause an increase in the severity of an already existing gingivitis. If the patient practices adequate home care and scrupulous oral hygiene so that no local irritants are present, gingivitis will not occur. However, because of the patient's physical state, there is an inclination on the part of many patients to decrease the amount of care given to their mouth. In addition, many of these patients are placed on high carbohydrate diets and soft foods which tend to accumulate on the teeth. The systemic influence of pregnancy on the gingiva usually disappears at the termination of pregnancy or shortly after parturition. At this time it is easier for the patient to maintain good oral hygiene and the response to surface irritants is no longer exaggerated. In some instances, a blastomatoid or tumor-like mass develops on the gingiva, especially involving interdental papillae, and is referred to as a "pregnancy tumor." These are non-neoplastic lesions found in both men and women who are predisposed to the formation of exuberant granulation tissue. Thus, pregnancy tumors are, in effect, pyogenic granulomas and are the result of an exaggerated response of the gingiva to injury.

Gingivitis associated with premenopause and postmenopause is not generally characterized by hyperplasia of the gingiva as occurs in pregnancy or puberty gingivitis. Gingivitis associated with endocrine dysfunctions at the time of menopause is referred to as hormonal gingivitis.

Diabetes mellitus is not a specific cause of periodontal disease. However, diabetic patients, especially those with uncontrolled diabetes, appear to be more susceptible to the presence of local irritants. It is generally recognized that uncontrolled diabetes tends to affect the resistance of the individual to irritation and bacterial infection. Not infrequently these patients suffer from multiple periodontal abscesses. It is obvious that the treatment of periodontal disease in patients with uncontrolled diabetes must include the removal of all local irritating factors. The control of diabetes mellitus is in the province of a physician.

16

Another systemic factor capable of modifying the response of the tissue to irritation is dilantin sodium. This drug, which is used in the treatment of epileptics, provokes an exaggerated response of the gingiva to irritation resulting in gingival hyperplasia or enlargement. This type of hyperplastic gingivitis is often referred to as dilantin gingivitis. However, dilantin sodium per se does not produce gingivitis. From a practical standpoint there is little tendency for hyperplasia of the gingiva to occur if all local irritating factors are removed prior to the administration of dilantin sodium.

As mentioned previously, no systemic disease per se is responsible for the production of periodontal disease. However, debilitating diseases may alter the resistance of the periodontal structures so that existing local irritating factors may produce a more severe response to injury than might be expected from the degree of irritating factors present. Probably of even greater importance is the decreased inclination of debilitated patients to adequately take care of their mouths.

From the foregoing discussion of the etiologic factors of periodontal disease, it is obvious that the primary cause of periodontal disease is of local origin, i.e., periodontal disease is inflammatory in nature and is the reaction of the tissues to injury. It is local in origin in that it is initiated by surface irritants arising from poor oral hygiene, faulty dentistry, mouth-breathing, improper tooth-brushing, and other irritants. Furthermore, dysfunctional irritants may also contribute to the production of periodontal disease, and systemic influences may appreciably alter the response of the tissue to the irritants. This concept of the etiology of periodontal disease places the emphasis of the treatment and prevention of periodontal disease on the removal of surface and dysfunctional irritants.

CLASSIFICATION

The following classification of periodontal disease is one of the many which have been proposed. The classification is based upon obvious clinical findings in the various forms of periodontal disease and upon the concepts of the etiology of periodontal disease which have been enumerated previously. Inasmuch as the primary reaction of the tissues to injury is inflammatory in nature and not initially or solely degenerative, such terms as gingivosis and periodontosis have been eliminated.

Simple gingivitis

Necrotizing ulcerative gingivitis (NUG, Vincent's infection)

Hyperplastic gingivitis
    Simple hyperplastic gingivitis
    Hereditary gingival fibromatosis

Gingivitis modified by systemic factors
    Dilantin hyperplasia
    Puberty gingivitis
    Pregnancy gingivitis

Hormonal gingivitis
    Chronic desquamative gingivitis (gingivosis)
    Chronic atrophic senile gingivitis

Atrophic gingivitis

Periodontitis

GINGIVITIS

Simple Gingivitis

Acute or chronic inflammation of the gingiva may be due to the effects of poor oral hygiene and other local irritants. There is a generalized or localized alteration of the gingival color varying from shades of coral pink with bluish tinge (cyanosis) to bright red. In some instances, the inflammatory reaction is limited to the free gingival margin and is referred to as marginal gingivitis (Fig. 131). Some degree of gingival enlargement may be present but it is not exaggerated. The depth of the gingival crevice may be somewhat increased. Pain is not a common feature, but bleeding on slight pressure is common. Bleeding occurs as the result of small ulcerations in the wall of the crevice and is a significant factor in the detection of gingivitis in patients who complain of "pink toothbrush." Such a complaint is often the first and only complaint of patients with early gingival disease and therefore should be considered an important complaint. Soft debris, materia alba, calculus, food impaction, overhanging margins, and other irritants are present.

The histopathology of gingivitis is related to the response of the tissues to injury and thus is primarily a picture of inflammation.

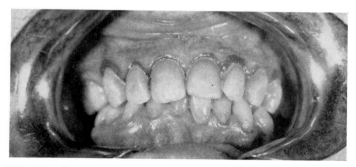

Figure 131. *Simple gingivitis.* Hyperemia of gingival margin of upper six anterior teeth.

Because of the chronicity of the irritating factors, the most common feature of simple gingivitis is active chronic inflammation. The color of the gingiva in simple gingivitis is related to vascular, connective tissue, and epithelial changes. Active hyperemia and a loss of keratinization, stippling, and the normal thickness of the epithelium account for areas of erythema. Impaired circulation and passive congestion (passive hyperemia) are responsible for the bluish tinge observed clinically. Inasmuch as active chronic inflammation is the most common finding in simple gingivitis, leukocytes and plasma cells are the most common inflammatory cells present. Inflammatory exudation and edema account for the spongy character of the gingiva in gingivitis. The normal architecture of the free gingival fibers may or may not be present, depending upon the character and duration of the inflammation. Varying degrees of epithelial proliferation and elongation of the rete pegs, especially of the gingival crevice, are generally present. It is common for the gingival crevice (crevicular epithelium) to show varying degrees of alteration. The loss of the continuity of the crevicular epithelium and the exposure of the underlying vascular bed of the granulation tissue present account for the ease of gingival hemorrhage. Gingival changes associated with acute inflammatory responses vary with the severity of the etiologic agent and the response of the tissues. In the absence of necrosis and/or ulceration, acute inflammatory changes are not common findings in simple gingivitis.

VINCENT'S INFECTION.   Pseudomembranous ulcerative necrotizing gingivitis (trench mouth) is an infective gingivitis associated with a fusospirochetal microorganism complex that becomes pathologic only after the vitality of the tissues has become impaired in some manner. While fusiform bacilli and spirochetes of Vincenti are always associated with necrotizing gingivitis, these organisms cannot be considered as primary etiologic agents in the causation of necrotizing gingivitis since more than 90 percent of the adult population have these organisms in their mouths continually. Although necrotizing gingivitis in the past was considered to be contagious, the consensus of present opinion and investigation indicates that Vincent's infection is transmissible but not communicable. Transmissible means that the infective stages of necrotizing gingivitis can be maintained through a susceptible host under experimental conditions. While necrotizing gingivitis may occur in individuals living in close approximation, its occurrence under such conditions should not be construed as evidence of contagiousness but rather that of a common environment predisposing to a decrease in the vitality of the tissues in susceptible individuals. Inasmuch as it is extremely difficult to grow Vincent's organisms outside the mouth, their survival on spoons, forks, and drinking glasses is problematical especially if the utensils are dried and exposed to the air as they usually are. In many instances, the reports of large outbreaks of necrotizing gingivitis are in reality reports of herpetic gingivostomatitis which is contagious. Furthermore, necrotizing gingivitis is always associated with local irritants. Even when necrotizing gingivitis occurs in a relatively clean mouth in one or two isolated areas, certain amounts of materia alba, plaque, or calculus are always found in such areas. While systemic factors which modify the vitality of the tissues appear to be important, the relationship of surface irritants and necrotizing gingivitis is even more important from a treatment standpoint inasmuch as the cure of acute necrotizing gingivitis is related to the removal of these irritants. Any symptomatic treatment, such as the use of antibiotics, that does not consider the complete removal of surface irritants results in a recurrence of the disease.

Although the inciting cause of necrotizing gingivitis is unknown, the following predisposing factors are important: poor oral hygiene, local irritants such as overhanging restorations, food impaction, excessive use of tobacco, erupting teeth, third molar tissue flaps, loss of sleep, and low tissue resistance from any disturbance in general metabolism.

The signs and symptoms of necrotizing gingivitis may be grouped according to the severity and duration of the disease. On this basis necrotizing gingivitis may be acute, subacute, or chronic in nature. The signs and symptoms of *acute* necrotizing gingivitis are as follows:

Sudden onset of "sore mouth"
Sloughing—necrosis mainly of the interdental papilla
Gray pseudomembrane with an erythematous border
Spontaneous bleeding
Odor—distinctive, foul fetid odor
Pain—gingiva extremely sensitive to touch
Increased salivation—metallic taste
Wedging sensation between teeth
Varying degrees of general symptoms such as malaise, fever, anorexia
Regional lymph node enlargement

Acute Vincent's infection is characterized by a sudden onset of a "sore mouth" wherein the patient complains of an extremely painful and sensitive gingiva which interferes with normal mastication. In some instances, patients will complain of fever, loss of appetite, and a general feeling of malaise. Slight pressure on the gingiva in an area of necrosis results in bleeding. Not infrequently patients will complain of a metallic taste and a wedging sensation around the teeth. The characteristic lesion of acute necrotizing gingivitis is the necrosis of the gingiva, mainly of the interdental papilla, which results in a marginated punched-out, eroded, and crater-like depression of the interdental papilla (Fig. 132). The surface of the lesion of necrotizing gingivitis is formed by a gray pseudomembranous slough demarcated from the remaining gingiva by an erythematous border. The pseudomembrane is removed easily and leaves a red, bleeding, ulcerated area. The teeth are generally covered by a soft mucinous plaque, especially in areas of active necrosis.

The term "subacute" is used to describe the type of necrotizing gingivitis in which the clinical signs and symptoms are less severe than in the acute form of the disease. All of the signs and symptoms of acute necrotizing gingivitis usually are not present in subacute Vincent's infection: the tissue involved may be limited to a few areas of the mouth; the destruction of tissue and pain are less severe; and the odor is not so overwhelming as in acute necrotizing gingivitis. The other symptoms, increased salivation, wedging sensation of the teeth, and constitutional symptoms, are generally minimal or absent. As in the acute form, lymph node enlargement may or may not be present.

The term "chronic necrotizing gingivitis" or "chronic Vincent's infection" is sometimes used to describe the effects of recurrent attacks of acute necrotizing gingivitis. The clinical features of "chronic Vincent's" are related to the destruction of the tissue and the reaction of the periodontium to previous attacks of acute or subacute necrotizing gingivitis. The histopathologic features of chronic Vincent's infection vary little from those often present in chronic destructive periodontal disease. Thus, in the absence of a previous

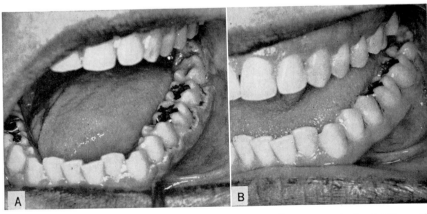

Figure 132. A, *Vincent's infection.* Necrotizing lesions typical of Vincent's infection at gingival margin of all posterior teeth B, Same areas as A following treatment.

history of "trench mouth," sore mouth, and Vincent's infection, the diagnosis of chronic Vincent's infection may be difficult to make. However, certain clinical features are suggestive of recurrent attacks of acute necrotizing gingivitis. The signs of recurrent episodes of acute and subacute necrotizing gingivitis are the presence of pseudopapilla, loss of interproximal tissue (punched-out interdental areas), and formation of gingival ledges associated with the loss of interdental papilla.

The histopathologic features of acute necrotizing gingivitis are those of a nonspecific necrotizing inflammation of the gingiva and the presence of a pseudomembrane. The surface of the lesion is composed of necrotic epithelium, polymorphonuclear leukocytes, fibrin, and microorganisms. This meshwork of necrotic debris appears clinically as the pseudomembrane and represents the effect of intercellular coagulation necrosis. At the borders and base of the lesion there is active hyperemia and infiltration of polymorphonuclear leukocytes. This response, as well as the thinning of the epithelium at the borders of the lesion, gives rise to the clinically apparent bright red border.

Hyperplastic Gingivitis

Hyperplastic gingivitis is a nonspecific inflammatory hyperplasia of the gingiva in response to chronic irritation. Gingival enlargement is a common feature of gingival disease and may involve any portion or all of the gingiva. Although some degree of gingival hyperplasia is common to all gingivitis, the term hyperplastic gingivitis is usually reserved to indicate a marked proliferative response of the gingiva.

SIMPLE HYPERPLASTIC GINGIVITIS. This form of gingivitis involves a marked proliferative response of the gingiva due to chronic irritation. It is characterized by nonspecific enlargement of the gingiva with clinical evidence of chronic irritants, such as calculus, soft debris, overhanging margins of restorations, and other local irritants, but no historical evidence of a systemic factor modifying the gingival response. *Simple hyperplastic gingivitis* differs from *simple gingivitis* in that the gingival crevice is deepened significantly and there is pronounced enlargement of the gingiva (Fig. 133). The histopathologic changes are similar to simple gingivitis, but epithelial and connective tissue responses are more prominent and result in a significant increase in size of the gingiva. Aside from the increase in size which may be evident microscopically as well as clinically, the histologic features of this type of gingivitis cannot be differentiated from simple gingivitis or other forms of hyperplastic gingivitis.

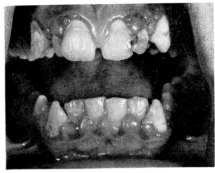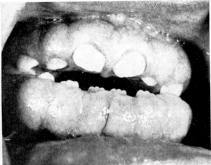

Figure 133. *Chronic simple hyper-plastic gingivitis.* There is marked thickening of gingival margin and increased bulk of interdental papillae in response to chronic irritation.

Figure 134. *Hereditary gingival fibromatosis.* Note malocclusion due to extensive gingival enlargement during and following eruption of the teeth.

HEREDITARY GINGIVAL FIBROMATOSIS.   This is a progressive proliferative response of the gingiva that appears to have hereditary or familial implications. The clinical aspects of this type of gingival disease include a diffuse enlargement of the gingiva which may be extensive enough to cover the surfaces of the teeth (Fig. 134). The gingiva is dense and firm and generally pale pink in color except in areas of active chronic inflammation. Enlargement of the gingiva may start with the eruption of the teeth in childhood or may not appear until adolescence. If the tissue is removed surgically, it usually reappears as the child grows older. A persistent progressive gingival enlargement and a positive familial history of this type of gingival enlargement are suggestive of hereditary gingival fibromatosis. However, when a history of familial incidence is lacking, the clinical picture may be confused with other forms of gingival enlargement. The persistent progressive enlargement of the gingiva, even where local factors are minimized, suggests the nature of the gingivitis. The histopathologic features responsible for the clinical appearance of gingival enlargement are a heavy overgrowth of subepithelial connective tissue. The connective tissue shows many well-defined, enlarged fiber bundles with only a relatively few blood vessels present. Superimposed inflammatory changes are present also. The microscopic features are relatively nonspecific and a definitive diagnosis of gingival fibromatosis can only be made in the presence of an adequate history and clinical examination.

Hyperplastic Gingivitis with Modifying Factors

The normal response of the gingiva to injury may be altered at the time of puberty or pregnancy and in association with the use of dilantin sodium. In no sense can pregnancy, puberty, or dilantin sodium administration be considered to be the primary cause of the gingivitis. The inflammation of the gingiva represents a response of the gingival tissues to irritation and injury. The exaggerated proliferative response of the tissues resulting in gingival enlargement can be attributed to the hormonal imbalance at the time of puberty or pregnancy and to the specific action of dilantin sodium, which is used in the treatment of epilepsy.

DILANTIN GINGIVITIS. This gingivitis is a progressive proliferative response of the gingiva associated with the use of dilantin sodium in the presence of local and dysfunctional irritants (Fig. 135). The enlargement of the gingiva associated with the use of dilantin sodium is nonspecific in character, and the degree of enlargement varies with an individual's response to the drug. The presence of teeth and local irritants appear to be prerequisites for gingival overgrowth, since gingival enlargement does not occur if the local irritants are removed prior to the institution of dilantin

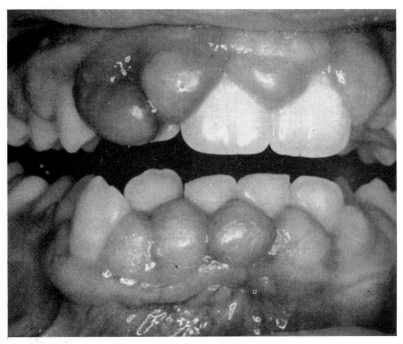

Figure 135. *Dilantin gingivitis.*

therapy and good oral hygiene is maintained. The proliferative potentialities of the gingiva in children and young adults appear to be greater than those of older individuals. The histopathologic features of dilantin gingivitis are those of a nonspecific inflammatory hyperplasia which cannot be distinguished microscopically from simple hyperplastic gingivitis.

PREGNANCY GINGIVITIS. The clinical features of pregnancy gingivitis do not differ from other forms of nonspecific inflammatory hyperplasia of the gingiva. The diagnosis of pregnancy gingivitis is made only on the basis of the physical state of pregnancy. In a relatively few individuals, a blastomatoid tumor-like lesion may involve the interdental papilla (Fig. 136). As mentioned previously, these lesions are merely an exaggerated response of the tissues to injury and represent an overgrowth of granulation tissue whose morphologic and histologic features are those of a granuloma pyogenicum. While pregnancy gingivitis cannot be considered to be a specific form of gingivitis related primarily to pregnancy, the altered response of the tissue to irritants at the time of pregnancy makes it mandatory that good oral hygiene be practiced at this time.

PUBERTY GINGIVITIS. This gingivitis is a nonspecific inflammatory hyperplasia of the gingiva initiated by local irritants and modified by hormonal stimulation at puberty. During puberty there often is an exaggerated gingival response to local irritation so that marked clinical changes occur as the result of even minimal surface irritants. The inflammatory response is usually severe resulting in a bluish-red discoloration of the gingiva, and gingival enlargement accompanied by diffuse edema resulting in very soft spongy tissues (Fig. 137). The alterations of color, form, and density of the gingiva may involve the entire mouth, but usually are more severe in the anterior portion of the mouth, especially in the presence of maloc-

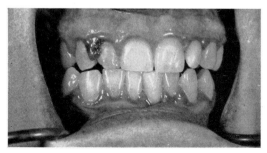

Figure 136. *Pregnancy gingivitis.* There is hyperemia and an increased bulk of the free gingival margin and interdental papillae. Focal enlargement between right lateral and cuspid is a so-called "pregnancy tumor."

clusion and mouth-breathing. There is some tendency for the gingival changes occurring at puberty to subside to some extent with the termination of puberty.

Hormonal Gingivitis

Hormonal gingivitis is a term used to describe certain forms of gingival disease in which the response of the tissues to local irritation is modified by sex hormones. A modification of the tissues' response to injury is not directed toward hyperplasia of the gingiva but rather to desquamative changes of the epithelium or to atrophy of the oral mucosa and gingiva. Hormonal gingivitis includes chronic desquamative gingivitis and chronic atrophic senile gingivitis.

CHRONIC DESQUAMATIVE GINGIVITIS. This type of gingivitis occurs primarily in females in association with an altered premenopausal hormonal stimulation. Periods of remission and exacerbations give rise to various clinical appearances of the gingiva. Varying degrees of severity may also be encountered. The patient's history usually indicates a gingivitis of long duration with remissions of short duration. Clinically, there is superficial desquamation of the epithelium and a tendency for the epithelium to become ulcerated easily (Fig. 138). Areas of pronounced desquamation of the epithelium and loss

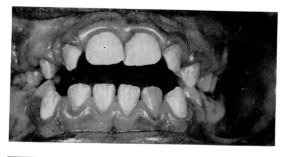

Figure 137. *Puberty gingivitis.* Increase in bulk and color of all gingival tissue in a patient about 13 years of age.

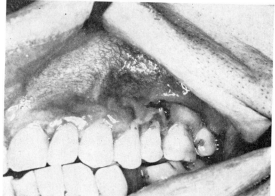

Figure 138. *Desquamative gingivitis.* Mottled area above bicuspids is produced by superficial necrosis and desquamation of gingival mucosa.

of stippling give the gingiva a somewhat patchy appearance. The color of the gingiva is generally reddish and the surface is smooth and glossy, especially in areas of active desquamation. Areas of erosion may be present leaving a painful, denuded, bleeding surface. Minor trauma, slight thermal change, and foods are not well tolerated. Patients with chronic desquamative gingivitis complain of a burning sensation in the mouth and extremely painful areas of the gingiva which have been denuded. The treatment of chronic desquamative gingivitis is directed toward the removal of irritation and trauma. However, a complete remission of the disease cannot be obtained as long as the altered premenopausal hormonal stimulation remains a factor. There are no specific histopathologic features that make diagnosis of desquamative gingivitis possible by microscopic means alone. The physical state of the patient and the clinical findings are also necessary to make a diagnosis. This form of gingivitis is sometimes called gingivosis.

CHRONIC ATROPHIC SENILE GINGIVITIS. Atrophic changes may develop in the gingiva and mouth following menopause. While these atrophic changes in the oral mucosa may occur during the menopause, the changes of atrophic senile gingivitis usually occur three to five years following menopause. This type of gingivitis is not common. The clinical features of the gingiva include gingival pallor, atrophy, and an inability of the oral mucosa to tolerate even minor traumatic injuries. The epithelial tissues are thin and atrophic, and there is little propensity of the gingiva and oral mucosa to adapt to even slight surface abrasion so that ulceration and bleeding occur frequently. Patients with this type of gingivitis do not tolerate dentures well because the atrophic epithelium does not respond to the presence of the denture by thickening the mucosa to accommodate the pressure. Burning sensations, dry mouth, and sensitivity to thermal changes and spicy foods are common complaints of individuals with senile atrophic gingivitis. Inasmuch as the oral mucosa of these patients does not respond well to surface and dysfunctional irritants, it is important that good oral hygiene be maintained and appliances be fitted as well as possible.

Atrophic Gingivitis

This type of gingivitis is characterized by gingival recession excessive for the age of the individual (Fig. 139). Clinically, the gingiva is usually relatively free of inflammation unless the exposed cementum is hypersensitive and for this reason the teeth are not kept clean. In many instances, the gingiva recedes at a rate equal to the loss of alveolar bone so that no increase in the depth of the gingival crevice occurs. Such recession may be due to inadequate

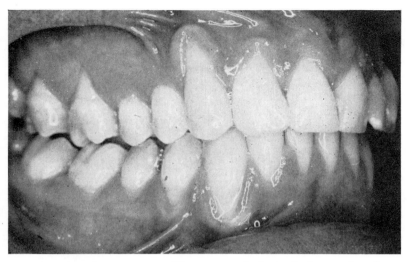

Figure 139. *Atrophic gingivitis.* There is marked gingival recession that may be due to gingival atrophy from the pressure of tooth-brushing or may be associated with trauma.

or improper tooth-brushing habits, hyperfunction, bruxism, or hypofunction. Generalized gingival recession involving the labial and buccal surfaces of the teeth occasionally may be present in young individuals and can be related to the unfavorable relationship produced by large teeth with inadequate bony support. Even though no increase in the depth of the crevice occurs with simultaneous apical migration of the epithelial attachment and recession of the free gingival margin below the cemento-enamel junction, such changes cannot be considered as physiologic regardless of the age of the patient. Thus, the concept of so-called physiologic recession, which involves simultaneous apical migration of the epithelial attachment below the cemento-enamel junction, atrophy of the gingival margin, simultaneous resorption of the alveolar crest, and compensatory eruption of teeth, cannot be considered as entirely valid, since etiologic factors responsible for gingival recession may always be found although their presence may be somewhat difficult to detect clinically.

PERIODONTITIS

Periodontitis is an inflammatory disease that is usually the sequelae of untreated gingivitis and is characterized by the extension of the inflammatory process into the deeper structures of the periodontium. The extension of the inflammation to the supporting structures of the teeth causes resorption of the alveolar bone, disor-

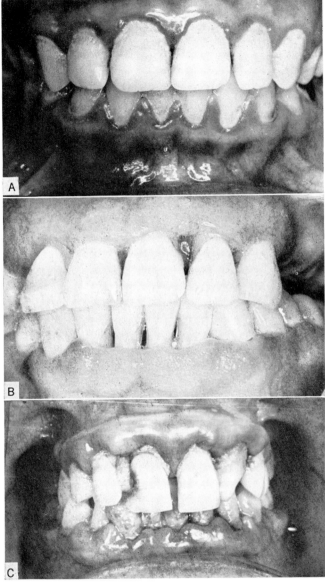

Figure 140. *Periodontitis.* A, Early periodontitis with marginal irritation associated with materia alba and subgingival calculus. Early pocket
formation could be demonstrated with a gingival probe. B, Advanced periodontitis with loss of interdental tissue suggesting
chronic Vincent's infection as an etiologic factor. C, Advanced
periodontitis with severe gingival reaction to poor oral hygiene
and to tooth mobility.

ganization of the principal fibers and their detachment from the cementum, and apical migration of the epithelial attachment along the root of the tooth. The detachment of the principal fibers and the apical migration of the epithelial attachment lead to pathologic deepening of the gingival crevice and the formation of a periodontal pocket. If the disease is not arrested, the detachment of the periodontal fibers and the resorption of the alveolar bone lead to hypermobility of the teeth and eventually to loss of the teeth.

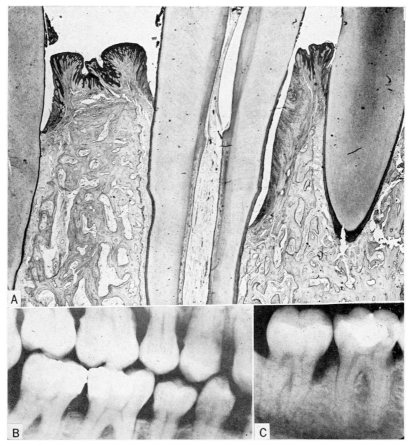

Figure 141. *Periodontitis.* A, Interproximal area on left shows horizontal pocket formation. The crevice in the interdental papillae is due to loss of free gingival fibers. Interdental area on right shows deep intrabony pocket. B, Radiograph showing loss of alveolar bone on all teeth. There is bifurcation involvement of lower molars. Note subgingival calculus on several root surfaces. C, Intrabony pocket on mesial side of lower second molar.

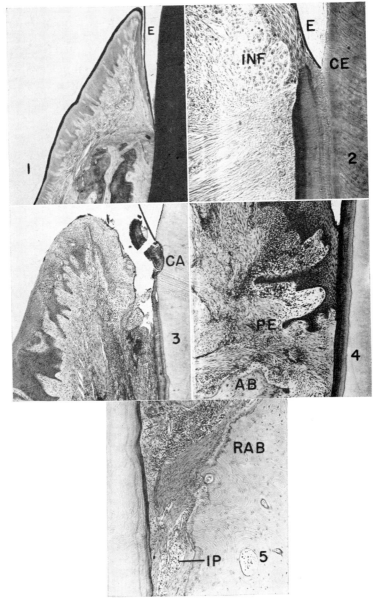

Figure 142. *Progress of periodontitis. Legend on opposite page.*

Periodontitis is manifested clinically by varying degrees of gingivitis with alterations in the color, form, and density of teeth reflecting the severity and chronicity of the inflammatory process in the periodontium (Fig. 140A, B, C). In order to determine the presence of periodontitis and periodontal pockets, it is necessary to probe carefully the depth of the entire gingival crevice with a thin periodontal probe. True periodontal pockets must be differentiated from gingival or relative pockets. An increase in the depth of the gingival crevice usually occurs in hyperplasia of the gingiva, i.e., hyperplastic gingivitis, even though the epithelial attachment is on the enamel. Such a pathologic deepening of the gingival crevice constitutes what is known as a relative, pseudo-, or gingival pocket. In contrast, if there is pathologic deepening of the gingival crevice, a loss of alveolar bone, and the base of the pocket (epithelial attachment) is on the cementum, such a deepening of the gingival crevice is said to be a true periodontal pocket.

The loss of alveolar bone associated with periodontitis may be seen radiographically by noting the lack of continuity of the lamina dura and the loss of height of the alveolar crest. The loss of supporting bone may be generalized or localized to individual teeth. An intrabony pocket is a periodontal pocket with the base of the pocket apical to the alveolar crest (Fig. 141A, C). It should be pointed out again that the presence of periodontal pockets can be determined accurately only by probing the gingival crevice with a thin periodontal probe.

The histopathologic features of periodontitis are those of a progressive inflammatory process (Fig. 142–1, 2, 3, 4, 5). The main features include the presence of a deepened gingival crevice (periodontal pocket) with its base or epithelial attachment on the cemen-

---

Figure 142. *Progress of periodontitis.* 1, Normal gingival attachment: space occupied by enamel, (E). 2, Early proliferation of epithelial attachment onto cementum and inflammatory infiltrations beneath crevicular epithelium: cemento-enamel junction, (CE); inflammatory infiltrations, (INF). 3, Moderately advanced periodontitis. The epithelial attachment is below the CE junction. An intense inflammatory reaction is present: calculus in depression at cemento-enamel junction, (CA). 4, Advanced periodontitis. The epithelial attachment is on the surface of cementum: proliferating epithelial attachment, (PE); alveolar bone, (AB). The mild inflammatory response at the base of the pocket is somewhat limited by epithelial proliferation. 5, Advanced periodontitis with spread of inflammation into the periodontal membrane and destruction of periodontal fibers with associated resorption of alveolar bone, (RAB). Spread of inflammation into interstitial areas of the periodontal membrane, (IP).

tum; loss of height of the alveolar crest; ulceration and proliferation of the epithelial lining of the pocket with underlying active chronic inflammation; loss of the functional arrangement of the periodontal fibers; and the presence of calculus on the cementum. The formation of a purulent exudate in chronic destructive periodontal disease reflects the nature of the inflammatory changes in the wall of the periodontal pocket.

The development of a periodontal pocket begins with gingivitis. Because of the presence of local irritants, especially supra- and subgingival calculus, the inflammatory reaction progressively involves the wall and base of the gingival crevice so that the epithelial lining of the gingival crevice becomes lost or ulcerated. The loss of the continuity of the gingival crevice epithelium provides an opening for the effects of bacterial toxins and enzymes. Bacterial enzymes, such as hyaluronidase, enhance the spread of bacterial toxins into the supporting structures. The continued presence of irritants and the progressive inflammatory response of the supporting structures lead to a resorption of the alveolar bone, loss of arrangement of the periodontal fibers, apical migration of the epithelial attachment, and a progressive deepening of the gingival crevice so that periodontal pockets are formed. The loss of alveolar bone and the detachment of the principal fibers of the periodontium and subsequent deepening of the periodontal pocket continue to occur as long as irritants such as calculus remain on the surfaces of the teeth.

Gingivitis and periodontitis represent reactions of the periodontium to injury. Reaction is primarily inflammatory in nature and is initiated principally by surface irritants. Thus, these diseases can largely be prevented by keeping the teeth free of calculus, plaque, and soft debris.

SEQUELAE OF PERIODONTITIS. When periodontitis is not arrested, alveolar bone continues to be lost to a point where the teeth do not have enough support to resist occlusal stresses, especially forces in a lateral direction. The loss of support leads to mobility and drifting of the teeth impairing their functional capacity and adding further injury to the already overburdened supporting structures. Ultimately such teeth may become so mobile as to require their extraction.

An extensive loss of alveolar bone occurring as the result of periodontitis leaves much to be desired of the remaining alveolar ridge as a base for partial and complete dentures (Fig. 143). Extension of periodontitis may, and often does, involve the bifurcation and trifurcation (interradices) areas of teeth (Fig. 144). The extension of periodontal pockets into interradicular areas makes treatment difficult, if not impossible, and extraction necessary.

Deepened gingival crevices associated with periodontitis are conducive to the formation of calculus and bacterial colonies and the ingress of foreign objects such as seeds, toothbrush bristles, and food fragments into the sulcus. These irritants frequently lead to injury and ulceration of the epithelial lining of the deepened gingi-

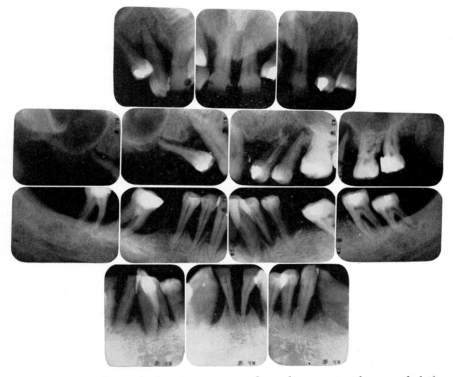

Figure 143. Radiograph showing extensive loss of supporting bone and drifting of teeth, the end result of long-standing periodontal disease. An extreme loss of bone jeopardizes the wearing of dentures.

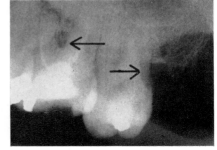

Figure 144. Radiograph showing trifurcation involvement of upper first and second molars.

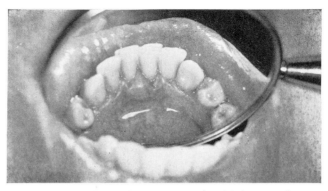

Figure 145. *Periodontal abscess* on lingual side of left central incisor.

val crevices and to the formation of periodontal abscesses (Fig. 145). A periodontal abscess is a local accumulation of pus in the periodontal tissues giving rise to a painful swelling. Drainage of the pus may occur spontaneously or require the use of probing instruments. Periodic swelling and spontaneous drainage with relief of pain may occur. Adequate treatment includes drainage and removal of the injurious agents.

BIBLIOGRAPHY

Ash, M. M.: Physiology of the mouth. In R. W. Bunting (Ed.): *Oral Hygiene.* Philadelphia, Lea & Febiger, 1957.

Kerr, D. A.: Classification and terminology for 1951 periodontal workshop. J. Amer. Dent. Ass., *44*:621, 1951.

Kerr, D. A.: Summary of systemic relations in periodontal disease. J. Periodont., *22*:27, 1951.

Kerr, D. A., Ash, M. M., and Millard, H. D.: *Oral Diagnosis,* 3rd ed. St. Louis, C. V. Mosby Co., 1969.

Kerr, D. A., Ramfjord, S. R., and Ash, M. M. (Eds.): World Workshop of Periodontal Disease. Ann Arbor, Mich., The Univ. of Mich. Press, 1966.

Marshall-Day, C. D.: The epidemiology of periodontal disease. J. Periodont., *22*:13, 1951.

Marshall-Day, C. D., Stevens, R. G., and Quigley, L. F., Jr.: Periodontal disease, prevalence and incidence. J. Periodont., *26*:185, 1955.

McIntosh, W. G.: Gingival and periodontal disease in children. Canad. Dent. Ass. J., *20*:12, 1954.

Ramfjord, S.: Local factors in periodontal disease. J. Amer. Dent. Ass., *44*:647, 1952.

Stomatitis is a broad term which includes all of the inflammatory processes involving the soft tissues of the oral cavity. Although it logically would include all of the inflammatory processes which occur in the gingiva, those involving the gingiva usually are excluded from the classification of stomatitis and placed under the separate heading of gingivitis. This placement is especially true of gingival disease that is limited to the free gingiva and is associated totally or in part with gingival irritation produced by accretions on the teeth and other local factors. Disease processes involving the gingiva concomitantly with other areas of the oral mucosa are classified as stomatitis. This procedure has been followed in this text, and the diseases unique to the gingiva are discussed in Chapter Eleven. This chapter includes inflammatory processes which involve one or more of the soft tissues and are due to mechanical, thermal, or chemical irritation, invasion by microorganisms, or to unknown causes. The various forms of stomatitis are discussed according to etiology and according to the changes which occur in the various anatomic locations. Because of the numerous possibilities of involvement in the various anatomic sites, the subject of stomatitis is extensive and utilizes more space than is commensurate with the scope of this text. Therefore, only the more common forms of stomatitis are included in this book.

TRAUMATIC STOMATITIS

Mechanical Injury

Because of the presence of hard structures such as the teeth and because of the motion produced by mastication of hard foods, mechanical injury to lips, buccal mucosa, and tongue is a frequent occurrence. One of the common forms of mechanical stomatitis is produced in the buccal and vestibular mucosa as the result of repeated or habitual cheek-biting. This type of injury is seen in individuals who have heavy jowls with thick buccal fat pads which press the buccal mucosa against the teeth. It is most likely to occur in the individual who has bruxism and in the patient who habitually chews the cheek as a nervous habit. The changes produced by cheek-biting are seen in the buccal mucosa along the line of occlusion of the teeth extending from the most posterior teeth to the commissure and just inside the vermilion border of the upper and lower lips. The character and distribution of the changes are dependent upon the position of the teeth and the severity of the irritation. In individuals in whom the mucosa is closely adapted to the teeth but in whom habitual chewing does not occur, a soft linear fold extends from the most posterior tooth to the commissure along the line of occlusion. The fold is indented in the area contacted by the teeth and conforms to the spaces between the teeth. The surface of the fold is slightly hyperkeratinized resulting in a mild opacity of the epithelium which gives a grayish-white appearance to the fold. This whitish linear fold at the line of occlusion is called *linea alba buccalis.*

In patients who exhibit bruxism, the mucosa may be trapped between the teeth producing small perforating or abrasive wounds (Fig. 146). The wounds often produce hemorrhage of a slight degree so that petechiae may be associated with the linea alba. In more severe cheek-chewing, the mucosa shows a more severe hyperkeratosis; it is grayish-white and shaggy and has irregular small erosions where the superficial layers of the mucosa have been stripped away by being grasped between the teeth while the cheek is pulled away. These tears may involve the full thickness of the mucosa and small ulcers result. In those cases where the habit is persistent, the surface mucosa is firm due to heavy keratinization and is opaque, white, and fissured. The underlying tissue is composed of scar, producing a firmness to the entire lesion. When the habit is vicious, the center of the lesion may be ulcerated and sore.

Changes due to mechanical injury of a chronic nature may also be seen in the lateral border of the anterior two-thirds of the tongue.

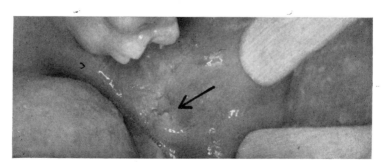

Figure 146. *Cheek-biting.* Arrow indicates destruction of buccal mucosa from biting. The depression is partially surrounded by a fold of scar.

In the patient with a tongue larger than can be accommodated in the arch of the mandibular teeth or in the patient who habitually presses the tongue against the teeth, lateral indentations following the contours of the teeth are produced. On rare occasions the pressure may be severe enough to produce hyperplastic changes consisting of grayish-white folds of the lateral border of the tongue which follow the contour of the teeth. Heavy folds with areas of ulceration rarely occur in the tongue owing to its more sensitive character which prevents the development of a habit vicious enough to produce extensive injury.

The lips may be irritated by contact with irregular, sharp anterior teeth or by habitual chewing (Fig. 147). The changes are the same as those present in the buccal mucosa. In patients, especially children, who have had nerve block anesthesia of the mandible resulting in numbing of the lip, a severe acute injury may result because of biting. The lip may be bitten several times with sufficient severity to perforate the tissues of a confined area. This results in a marked swelling with numerous small ulcers which become confluent to produce a large single ulcer. The tissue fluid exuding from the ulcer produces a heavy crust on the vermilion border. The acute swelling and crusting of one-half or more of the lower lip are alarming to the patient or parent, but the history of a sudden occurrence

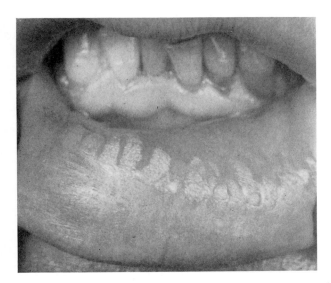

Figure 147. *Focal hyperkeratosis.* The white verrucal elevations in the vestibular mucosa are slightly firmer than the surrounding mucosa. The white, firm character is the result of hyperkeratosis produced by smoking and by rubbing the tissue against sharp upper teeth.

following local anesthesia is characteristic and indicates the traumatic character of the lesion.

Similar changes may be produced by contact with sharp teeth or denture clasps. In this situation the lesions are localized to the small area adjacent to the rough tooth or clasp producing the injury. In the retromolar area, limited space may be available to accommodate the third molars, resulting in their malposition which predisposes to impingement of the buccal mucosa or gingival flaps overlapping the molars. These areas of impingement frequently become sore and ulcerated due to swelling which enhances the impingement.

Mechanical injury is frequently produced in the gingiva owing to the vigorous use of a stiff toothbrush. The onset of tenderness is rather rapid and is due to the presence of multiple small ulcers of circular or linear configuration (Fig. 128). The stiff bristles of the brush either perforate or lacerate the gingiva, depending upon the method of application. The lesions are most severe at the height of contour of the gingiva over the roots of the teeth and at the gingival margins. They may occur on the labial, buccal, palatal, or lingual aspects of the gingiva. Tooth-brushing abrasion may be bilateral, and if so, it is most intense on the side opposite to the hand holding the brush. Toothbrush injury is accompanied by a burning type of tenderness of the entire area involved. The ulcers heal in three to five days if the injury is not repeated.

Mechanical injury also occurs under dentures, especially upper dentures which occlude against all natural teeth or against a few natural teeth and a partial denture. This type of injury occurs most frequently under areas of abnormal denture pressure on the anterior maxillary ridge and the vault of the palate. In the anterior ridge area the tissue becomes red, swollen, and flabby (Fig. 50). The tissue has a tendency to be thrown into folds and may be crowded over the labial flange of the denture. In the palatal area the tissue becomes intensely red, smooth, and tender. There is hyperplasia of a polypoid character which produces a pebbly or cauliflower appearance to the surface.

Thermal Injury

Thermal irritation is usually produced by taking hot foods into the mouth. The degree and location of the burn depend on the type and temperature of the food. If the food is fluid, the burn occurs on the anterior one-third of the tongue and the anterior palate. If the food is semi-solid and adheres to the tissue, the burn area is more localized and intense. The change in the tongue is usually redness, especially of the papillae. In the palate the area posterior to the incisors is red and swollen. In the areas where

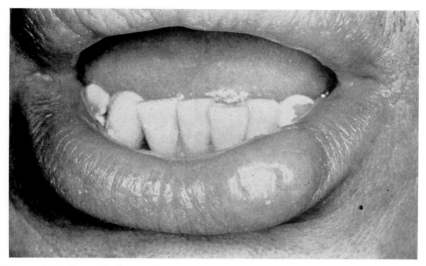

Figure 148. *Second degree burn.* The large vesicle on the lower lip was produced by the anesthetized lip contacting a hot hydrocolloid
syringe.

hot, sticky material contacts the tissue, the burn is localized and
superficial ulcers follow vesiculation (Fig. 148). The vesicles rupture
almost as soon as they are formed and therefore are rarely observed.
Thermal burns may be produced by the introduction of hot impression materials and are localized in the area contacted by the material. They are of variable severity depending upon the temperature of the material.

Chemical Injury

Various chemical substances due to either repeated or prolonged
contact may produce irritation of the oral mucosa. Mild change may
be produced by dentifrices containing strong flavoring or detergent
materials (Fig. 149). The changes are most marked in the buccal
mucosa and to a lesser degree in the floor of the mouth, but are
usually not produced in the area of the mucosa which is keratinized. The mucosal surface is covered by a thin slimy, grayish, slightly
opaque film which can be rubbed or peeled away. The membrane is
superficial and somewhat folded in appearance. When removed, the
underlying mucosa is of normal appearance. There are usually no
attendant symptoms, but the patient is aware of a slight burning
sensation when the dentifrice is used. A similar whitish appearance
may be produced by mouthwashes, especially those having a high
alcoholic content. When hydrogen peroxide is used persistently as

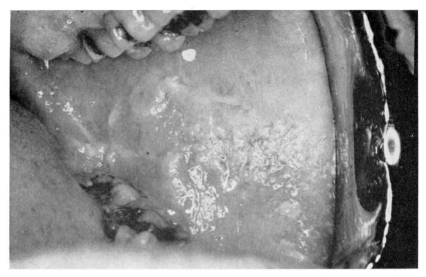

Figure 149. *Dentifrice reaction.* The superficial necrotic change in the buccal mucosa produces a friable, thin, opaque, gelatinous membrane which separates easily, providing a "peeling" effect. The change is due to the detergent in the dentifrice.

a mouthwash, it produces keratinization of the tongue with an accentuation of the filiform papillae, giving the tongue the appearance of being covered with a brown fur. The coating appears within a few days after starting to use hydrogen peroxide as a mouthwash and persists for some days after the practice is discontinued.

Mild chemical burns may be produced by the repeated application of "toothache drops" (Fig. 152). They produce redness in the area of application and may, with overzealous use, produce ulceration. The areas involved may be the lips, buccal mucosa, lateral border of the tongue, or gingiva. In mild burns the tissue is red, but with severe burns a whitish slough covers an intensely red zone which extends beyond the border of the slough. Chemical burns may be produced by the intentional or accidental application of caustic agents to the mucosa. Silver nitrate (Fig. 150), phenol (Fig. 151), trichloroacetic acid, zinc chloride and "toothache drops" (Fig. 152) are all examples of agents which may be used by doctor or patient. Aspirin burns are frequently produced by patients holding aspirin tablets in contact with the mucosa for pain relief (Fig. 153). Strong acids, alkalies and oxidizing agents in mild to strong concentrations produce destruction of mucosa. The accidental ingestion of lye, by children, results in severe destructive chemical injury.

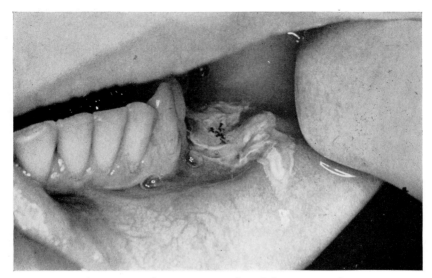

Figure 150. *Silver nitrate burn.* Burn produced large area of necrotic mucosa and fibrinous membrane in the mucobuccal fold. Black material in the center is precipitated silver.

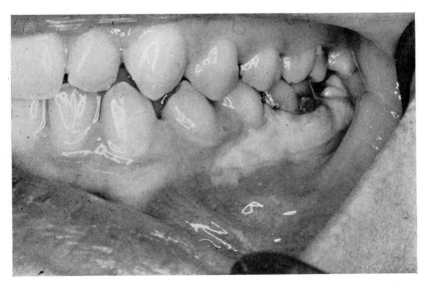

Figure 151. *Phenol burn.* Intercellular coagulation necrosis of gingival tissue below the bicuspids and the first molar caused by burn. The coagulated area is opaque, grayish white in appearance.

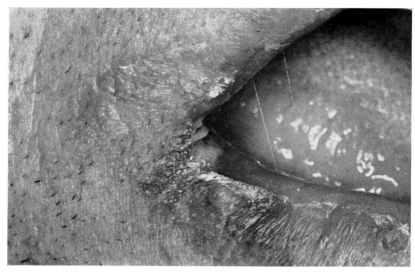

Figure 152. *Chemical burn* (from toothache drops). The burn involves the angle of the mouth and the lower lip almost to the midline. It also involves the lateral aspect of the tongue. The intensity of the burn varies from erythema on the tongue to necrosis at the angle of the mouth.

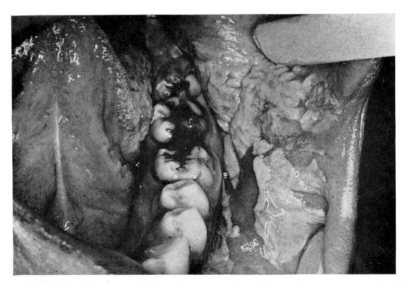

Figure 153. *Aspirin burn.* Extensive necrosis of buccal mucosa and slight necrosis on the posterior lateral border of the tongue opposite the second bicuspid and first molar caused by aspirin. The membrane has separated from the regenerated mucosa. The pericoronitis about the last molar was the reason for holding aspirin in the area.

Chemical irritation may be produced by smoking or chewing tobacco. In smoking the changes are produced in the palate, buccal mucosa, and the tongue. They occur initially in the palate and are limited to the palate except in severe cases. When the changes are mild and early the palate is pale, especially the posterior two-thirds. The orifices of the palatal glands appear as red pinpoint perforations. These changes are due to hyperkeratinization and hyperplasia of the palatal epithelium and slight dilatation of the duct orifice. When the process is more severe and of a more chronic nature, the palate is whiter and numerous papules (1 to 2 millimeters in diameter) appear on the surface (Fig. 154). The papular structure appears in the midline of the posterior one-half or one-third of the palate. The elevations have red to pink punctate centers which mark the gland orifice. In very severe cases the papular lesions may be close together and produce a pattern of fissuring. When the smoking is intense and of long duration, the buccal mucosa and tongue become grayish-white and leathery owing to hyperkeratinization. In edentulous patients the hyperkeratinization of the alveolar ridge and buccal mucosa have a sharp line of demarcation at the point of contact and the hyperkeratinization does not extend into the buccal fornix.

The changes produced by the use of chewing tobacco or snuff are those of hyperkeratinization and hyperplasia in the area contacted by the tobacco. The tissue is grayish-white in color and slightly folded or wrinkled. In persons who use chewing tobacco, the changes are in the buccal mucosa of the buccal pouch and involve the gingiva. In individuals using snuff, the alteration is usually in the anterior mucobuccal fold on either side of the mid-

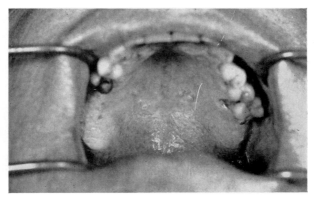

Figure 154. *Nicotine stomatitis.* Small papillomatous areas produced by dilatation of ducts of accessory salivary glands with metaplasia of ductal epithelium. Whitish appearance of palate is due to hyperkeratosis.

line and involves gingival and vestibular mucosa of a very limited area because the individual habitually holds the snuff in the same location. Continuous use of chewing tobacco or snuff over protracted periods of time results in very intense changes, and a warty appearance of the lesions suggests the development of a verrucal carcinoma. Verrucal carcinoma is a particular type of carcinoma resulting from the prolonged use of tobacco.

STOMATITIS DUE TO MICROORGANISMS

A variety of changes may be produced in the oral mucosa by microorganisms, and the changes produced are usually quite characteristic for each variety of organism. The resulting disease is usually designated by the causative organism. The herpes simplex virus produces two forms of stomatitis; one as the result of the initial invasion of the virus designated *primary herpetic gingivostomatitis,* the second a recurrent process secondary to the initial infection designated *recurrent herpetic stomatitis,* chronic habitual aphthae, or chronic recurrent aphthous stomatitis.

PRIMARY HERPETIC GINGIVOSTOMATITIS.   This disease is produced by initial infection with the herpes simplex virus and is a generalized disease involving the oral mucosa, the gingiva, the regional lymph nodes, and the lymphoid tissue of the pharynx and sometimes the skin. The herpes simplex virus is a very common organism easily transmitted from one person to another so that 90 percent of the adult population have antibodies in their sera indicating previous infection. Infection is most common in early life with the highest incidence between the ages of two and five years. The disease has

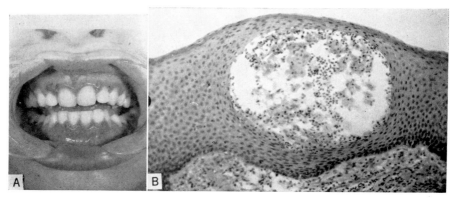

Figure 155. *Herpetic gingivostomatitis.* A, There is extensive hyperemia and swelling of free gingiva with small ulcer above the right lateral incisor resulting from ruptured vesicle. B, Intraepithelial vesicle of the type present in herpetic gingivostomatitis.

a sudden onset with high fever, painful swollen submaxillary lymph nodes, and sore throat. After 48 hours the mouth becomes sore owing to changes in the gingiva and mucosa. The gingiva becomes red, swollen, and tender. The mucosa is red and tender and one to several small vesicles appear. They are thin-walled and rupture easily, leaving a superficial ulcer which rapidly becomes covered with a fibrinous membrane (Fig. 155). The membrane is yellowish in color, firmly adherent, and is surrounded by a very red inflammatory halo or border about 1 millimeter in width (Fig. 156). The ulcer becomes very painful. With the appearance of the vesicles the temperature drops to nearly normal. The symptoms remain severe for a few days then gradually subside. The ulcers heal within 10 to 14 days, the gingiva returns to normal, and the lymphadenitis subsides. Mild lymphadenitis may persist for several weeks. During the later stages of the disease antibodies begin to build up in the blood serum. The antibody titer builds up for some weeks after the disease has subsided. The antibody titer of the blood reaches a high level and then subsides, but not completely. The persistent antibodies provide some protection and the individual never develops a second episode of primary herpetic gingivostomatitis but may have recurrent attacks of localized lesions. The recurrent attacks are called secondary herpetic stomatitis, recurrent habitual aphthae, or recurrent herpetic stomatitis. Individual lesions occurring on the lips are commonly referred to as "cold sores," whereas those within the mouth are called "canker sores." The lip lesions (herpes labialis or "cold sores") most often occur on the vermilion border but may occur on the circumoral skin (Fig. 157). They begin with a burning sensation and a swelling of the lip rapidly followed

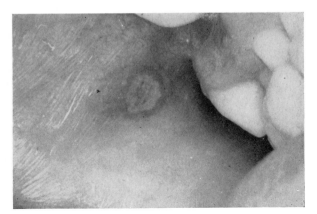

Figure 156. *Herpetic ulcer in buccal mucosa.* Note yellow membranous center with peripheral zone of hyperemia.

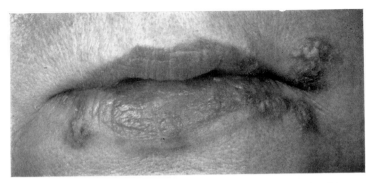

Figure 157. *Herpes labialis* (*"cold sore"*). Vesicular stage of cold sore. Note the numerous small vesicles which later coalesce to form a single lesion.

by an aggregate of small vesicles which have a tendency to coalesce then rupture and exude serum that forms an abundant yellowish crust. The lesions may crack with movement of the lip causing hemorrhage, and the crust becomes black in color. Herpes labialis usually heal in two or three weeks without residual scar. The lesions may recur at varying intervals, frequently in the same location. Following the initial infection the virus is residual in the tissue and may be activated by anything which lowers the resistance of the tissue. Some patients develop lesions following each dental appointment from trauma produced by the manipulation of the lip. Some individuals develop lesions following exposure to sunlight. The lesions are associated with upper respiratory infection or other disease processes attended by a fever, and, for this reason, the lesions are referred to as fever blisters. Some patients associate them with gastrointestinal upsets in which case they are often due to food allergies. They may also be associated with the onset of menstrual periods. Treatment is symptomatic as the lesions heal spontaneously. The lesions should be kept soft by the application of cold cream, petroleum jelly, or an ointment with a lanolin base. Secondary infection is rarely a problem and therefore antiseptic ointments are not necessary.

Herpetic lesions may be aborted if treated when the initial symptoms appear and before vesiculation is evident. This can be done on the lips by the application of dehydrating agents to the area as soon as the patient is aware of the initial burning sensation and swelling. Absolute alcohol and ether in equal parts applied to the area every few minutes for one or two hours or until the symptoms subside will abort the lesion. It may be aborted in some instances by the application of an ointment containing hydrocortisone acetate when the initial symptoms appear.

Canker sores (aphthous ulcers, herpetic ulcers) are recurrent herpetic lesions involving mucous membrane. They occur in vestibular and buccal mucosa, floor of the mouth, the gingiva, and on the tongue. Those occurring in the mucobuccal fold are linear in shape and are called aphthous fissuratum, while those in other areas are round or oval and are called canker sores. The initial symptoms are not as pronounced as the lesions on the lip, and the patient may not be aware of the onset of the lesion. As on the lip, the lesion arises as a vesicle but, owing to its location on a moist non-keratinized surface, the vesicle ruptures easily and is therefore present for only a very short time and the vesicular state is not recognized by the patient. After the vesicle ruptures, a shallow ulcer develops which is rapidly covered by a yellowish fibrinous membrane surrounded by an intense red zone 1 or 1½ millimeters in width. The ulcer becomes very painful, especially when it is located in the areas where the tissue is movable. The lesions may be single or multiple and of variable size, some reaching 5 to 7 millimeters in diameter. The pain is usually more intense when the lesions are large and multiple. The lesions heal spontaneously in seven to 14 days. Treatment is valuable only to relieve pain and does not enhance healing. Pain may be relieved by the application of Xylocaine (viscous) for a short period to permit the patient to eat more comfortably. Very painful ulcers may be relieved by chemical cautery of the base of the lesion. The lesions may be initiated by menstruation, food allergies, local trauma, and upper respiratory infections. They may be prevented by the use of immune gamma globulin serum, smallpox vaccine, and other means associated with a specific predisposing factor, such as menstruation, allergy, or emotional tension.

Other forms of infectious stomatitis are rare but may occur in association with disease processes in other areas of the body. Secondary syphilitic lesions may occur in the oral mucosa and resemble the aphthous ulcer, except that they are usually not painful and do not have distinct inflammatory halos. Patients with pulmonary tuberculosis may develop tuberculous ulcers of the oral mucosa. They are usually small crater-form ulcers having a brownish, gelatinous, membranous base. The ulcers are very painful and have no tendency for healing. The history of pulmonary tuberculosis is usually obtained, but in some instances pulmonary disease may be unrecognized.

ACTINOMYCOSIS. This is a disease involving the jaws and is caused by a fungi (actinomyces). In this disease, abscesses are

18

formed which rupture into the oral cavity or through the skin to produce a draining sinus. Often multiple sinuses are present with intermittent drainage of pus containing yellowish granules. The organisms appear to enter the tissue through some surface defect, such as an open extraction site or a periodontal pocket. A similar disease, "lumpy jaw," is present in cattle and other domestic animals and is suggested as the source of infection in man although it is seen in many individuals having no contact with farm animals.

CANDIDIASIS (THRUSH).   Candidiasis is an infection produced by a yeast (Candida albicans). This infection usually occurs in the very young or very old, especially those debilitated by some other disease. It is also seen in individuals who have had intense prolonged antibiotic therapy. It involves the pharynx and oral mucosa producing irregular reddish zones with multiple shallow ulcers covered by a white friable membrane (Fig. 158). The membrane is loosely adherent and leaves a shallow and tender but not painful ulcer when removed. The presence of numerous, slightly elevated, white flecks spread over the erythematous mucous membrane and resembling curds of milk is typical of this infection.

STOMATITIS AND SYSTEMIC DISEASE

Certain systemic diseases, especially those of dermatologic nature, may involve the oral mucosa. Only the most common oral manifestations of systemic diseases are discussed. The acute infectious diseases characterized by skin rash occasionally involve the oral mucosa in a characteristic fashion.

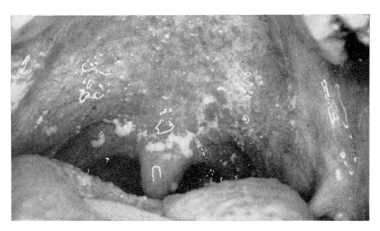

Figure 158. *Thrush (candidiasis)*. Irregular white patches resembling milk curd on soft palate and uvula.

EXANTHEMATOUS DISEASES. Chickenpox is an exanthematous disease which may produce oral lesions in large numbers. The lesions are vesicles similar to those of the skin but rupture rapidly due to the moist environment. The residual lesion is a superficial ulcer which heals at the same rate as the skin lesions.

In measles, during the second day of the prodromal phase, and about 24 hours before the appearance of the rash, Koplik's spots occur in the buccal mucosa along the line of occlusion. The patient first experiences a burning sensation of the area just before the development of a pinhead-sized, white or bluish spot surrounded by an inflamed red zone. The spots fade and gradually disappear as the mucosa increases in redness and the skin lesions appear. The presence of Koplik's spots, with the accompanying fever, coryza, and photophobia, makes it possible to diagnose measles before the skin rash appears.

In scarlet fever characteristic lesions occur in the tongue. At first the tongue is heavily coated on the entire dorsum. The coating starts to disappear from the lateral border and progresses over the dorsum until the entire tongue is free of coating. As the coating disappears, the surface of the tongue appears studded with small elevated red dots which are the inflamed fungiform papillae. With complete loss of the coating, the tongue has a red, glazed appearance studded with red dots and is referred to as "strawberry tongue."

Oral Manifestations of Dermatologic Diseases

Dermatologic diseases may be manifest in the oral mucosa owing to the similar ectodermal origin of the skin and oral mucosa. Oral lesions are seen in such dermatoses as lichen planus, herpes zoster (shingles), pemphigus, lupus erythematosus and some of the more rare skin diseases. Lichen planus involves the oral mucosa much more frequently than other forms of dermatoses and is the only one to be discussed here.

LICHEN PLANUS. This disease may involve the oral mucosa concomitantly with skin lesions or it may occur without skin involvement. All parts of the oral mucosa may be involved but the most frequent site is the buccal mucosa of the retromolar region. In some instances the tongue and/or gingiva may be involved. The severity of involvement of the various areas is not uniform. In one instance the tongue may be most severely affected, whereas in another it may be the gingiva or the buccal mucosa. The lesions present different features in each area and therefore will be discussed separately.

The lesions of the buccal mucosa consist of fine, pearly gray lines (striae) which exhibit a branching pattern (Fig. 159). At the point

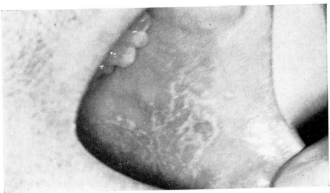

Figure 159. *Lichen planus.* Grayish-white striae producing a mesh-like pattern in the buccal mucosa are a characteristic but not a consistent finding in lichen planus.

where the striae cross, the lesion is slightly elevated and appears as a 1 millimeter grayish-white dot. The anastomosing striae produce a net-like pattern opposite to or posterior to the molar teeth. In some instances, where there is chronic irritation such as might be produced by a rough tooth or a dental appliance, the lesion becomes eroded. The erosion is superficial with a reddish base and is surrounded by the grayish-white mucosa.

In the tongue the striae are rare and the lesion is more plaque-like in character. The surface areas are grayish-white, slightly wrinkled, and there is atrophy of the papillae. Because of the very slight elevation of the lesion and its grayish color, the plaque form of lichen planus blends with the coating of the tongue and may be easily overlooked.

The gingival changes of lichen planus are of two types—the keratinized lesion and the erosive lesion. Erosion occurs in gingival involvement because of frequent irritation produced by chewing and by brushing the teeth. In the non-erosive form, the gingiva is grayish-white, wrinkled, and slightly firm; striae rarely appear. Lichen planus of the gingiva is frequently mistaken for focal hyperkeratosis or leukoplakia when the tongue and buccal mucosa are unaffected. The erosive lesion is painful, in contrast to the non-erosive type, in which the patient may be totally unaware of its presence. The gingiva is irregularly eroded providing a red and grayish mottled appearance. The erosion is superficial, red, and painful, while the other areas are grayish-white and non-tender. The pattern of erosion changes as one area heals and another becomes eroded. This condition is sometimes confused with chronic desquamative gingivitis.

ALLERGIC STOMATITIS

Allergic reactions may occur in the oral mucosa either as part of a generalized allergic response or as a local reaction owing to contact with dentifrices, cosmetics, and mouthwashes. The oral lesions associated with a generalized allergic response are most often due to sensitivity to drugs or foods (stomatitis medicamentosa). All drugs may produce an allergic response in some individuals, but the heavy metals (mercury, bismuth, lead, gold) and the antibiotics are the most frequent offenders. The allergic response is characterized by redness, soreness, mucosal necrosis, and ulceration which is not specific for any particular antigen. The lesions occur suddenly without apparent cause and become more severe as long as the drug is continued. When the drug is withdrawn, the lesions heal within a few days to a week. A history of the sudden occurrence of lesions without apparent cause (mottled areas of ulceration, redness, and tenderness) and the evidence that the patient is taking certain drugs suggest the diagnosis of an allergic stomatitis. Localized reactions in response to contact with drugs (stomatitis venenata) also may occur. Certain dentifrices, oil of cloves, oil of wintergreen, and other dental therapeutic agents may elicit an allergic response

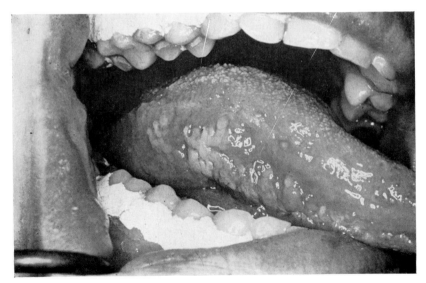

Figure 160. *Allergic response.* The grayish lesions on the lateral border of the tongue are areas of necrotic mucosa. The base of the lesion is intensely red. The allergic response occurs in all of the tissue contacting the surgical dressing which can be seen in place on both upper and lower jaws.

of redness and swelling (urticaria). Surgical dressings containing essential oils also may produce an allergic stomatitis (Fig. 160).

BIBLIOGRAPHY

Cawley, E. D., and Kerr, D. A.: Lichen planus. Oral Surg., 5:1069, 1952.
Kerr, D. A.: Herpetic gingivostomatitis. J. Amer. Dent. Ass., 44:674, 1952.

• Chapter 13
ENDOCRINE DISEASES

The substances produced by the endocrine glands (or ductless glands) are called hormones. Hormones are essential to many of the processes concerned with metabolism, growth, and reproduction. The principal hormone-producing organs are the pituitary, thyroid, parathyroids, adrenals, pancreas (islands of Langerhans), and the gonads. Many of the effects of endocrine functions are in balance due to an equilibria of the chemical reactions of the hormones and the nervous system. The hormonal regulation of body functions is accomplished by direct action on tissues, by influencing the secretion of other endocrine glands, and by acting on the nervous system. The brain must be considered an essential part of the complex mechanism of integrating hormonal influence on body functions since the hypothalamus is a center for the control of the anterior lobe of the pituitary gland, and since certain nuclei of the hypothalamus constitute an integral part of the neurohypophysis.

Certain hormones are tropic (trophic) in character; that is they act on another endocrine gland (target gland) and not directly on body cells. This is particularly true for the adrenals, thyroid, and gonads. The tropic hormone causes the target gland to produce its own hormone which then acts on the cells of the body tissues and, to some extent, in an inhibitory manner on the source of the tropic hormone. Thus, tropic hormones may be increased or decreased according to the output of the hormones on the target glands. Disturbances in the function of the endocrine glands may result in hypo- or hypersecretion of hormones and produce alterations in metabolism and growth. The age and state of body development of an individual are important in determining the effect these hormonal disturbances may have on the body.

Hormones are proteins, steroids, and amines of small molecular weight. Hormones that are protein in nature are secreted by the anterior pituitary, the parathyroids, the pancreas, and the thyroid glands. Steroid hormones are produced by the adrenal cortex, the testes, and ovaries. Amine hormones essentially are derived from cells of nervous origin, principally the neurohypophysis and the medulla of the adrenal gland.

Of particular interest is the role of the endocrines in healing wounds, especially healing of serious traumatic injuries or significant surgical procedures. In severe tissue damage certain hormones of the adrenal cortex, the adrenal medulla, and the posterior pituitary glands are important in the metabolic changes associated with the systemic effects secondary to the trauma or injury. Hormones influence the process of inflammation, repair, and regeneration in many ways. For example, it has been found that adrenal cortical extracts are capable of inhibiting the increase in capillary permeability associated with acute inflammation. Hydrocortisone, corticosterone, and cortisone tend to decrease inflammation, while desoxycorticosterone (DOC) and pituitary somatotropic hormone (STH) have the opposite effect. Injection of adrenocorticotropic hormone (ACTH) liberates hydrocortisone from the adrenal cortex, resulting in reduced capillary permeability, decreased exudation, and diminished formation of granulation tissue. There is also a decrease in lymphocytes in the circulating blood, and lymphocytic migration is inhibited following the administration of cortisone and ACTH. Although it has been said that cortisone inhibits phagocytosis, the evidence is contradictory. Hormonal influences on repair and healing of wounds are reflected in changes in connective tissue, viz., cortisone and ACTH inhibit wound healing by suppressive action on connective tissue proliferation. Histochemical studies indicate that acid mucopolysaccharides, chondroitin sulfate, hyaluronic acid, and collagen formation are diminished or depressed under the effect of cortisone. Also, large doses of estrogens appear to inhibit the formation of connective tissue. However, cortisone does not inhibit wound healing in therapeutic doses. Thus, the observations on hormonal influence of wound healing have a limited counterpart in clinical experience.

The effects of endocrine dysfunctions have been studied in patients with hyper- or hypofunctioning endocrine glands and in experimental animals subjected to injections of hormones and/or removal of endocrine glands. It should be remembered that dysfunction of one gland may be reflected in other glands as well.

PITUITARY DYSFUNCTION

The pituitary gland (hypophysis) is concerned with many vital processes, and at least ten hormones have been isolated from it. There is a reciprocal relationship between the pituitary gland and other endocrine glands as well as between the pituitary gland and the central nervous system. The pituitary gland has been called the master gland because of its influence on and control of the other endocrine glands. A characteristic function of the anterior portion of the pituitary gland is the elaboration of hormones which influence the activities of the other endocrine glands. Such hormones (tropic hormones) include the gonadotropic, thyrotropic, and adrenocorticotropic hormones.

The growth hormone or somatotropic hormone (STH) is not really a tropic hormone in that it does not produce its action by mediation on any target gland. It is necessary for growth and development and affects protein, fat, and carbohydrate metabolism. It should be pointed out that the growth hormone is relatively species-specific, viz., the bovine growth hormone produces little effect in man, while the growth hormone of monkeys may exert a significant anabolic effect on humans.

The adrenocorticotropic hormone (adrenocorticotropin, corticotropin, ACTH) is essential for the integrity of the adrenal cortex and stimulates the adrenal cortex to increase production of certain of the steroid hormones. The pituitary-adrenal relationship (pituitary-adrenal axis) is important in all kinds of nonspecific stress of physical, chemical, thermal, psychic, and bacterial origin. In effect, when the body is subjected to nonspecific stress, the anterior pituitary produces ACTH which in turn stimulates the adrenal cortex to produce corticosteroids. The relationship of ACTH and the adrenal mechanism acts to regulate in part all of the following: the mobilization of protein, the glucose level of the blood, the resorption of water and electrolytes in the renal tubules of the kidney, the amount of glycogen in the liver, the process of inflammation, the amount of lymphoid tissue, the integrity of the connective tissue, and some immune responses.

The thyrotropic hormone (thyrotropin, TSH) of the pituitary gland is necessary for maintenance of thyroid cells and stimulates the secretion of thyroid hormone. The effect of thyrotropic hormone is mediated not only by the amount of thyroid but probably also by the hypothalamus.

The principal causes of dysfunction of the pituitary gland include tumors arising in and near the gland, and to a lesser extent, lesions involving the blood vessels supplying the gland. Tumors arising from cells within the pituitary gland may result in an increased production of hormone or result in a reduction in the amount of hormone formed owing to pressure from the expanding lesions. Tumors of the pituitary gland may also result in hyperfunction and hyperplasia of the adrenal cortex, parathyroids, islets of Langerhans, and mammary glands.

Hypopituitarism

The most common organic cause of hypopituitarism is the craniopharyngioma, a tumor arising from remnants of the epithelial tract (craniopharyngeal duct) of Rathke's pharyngeal pouch. The *cranio-*

pharyngioma often has the characteristics of an ameloblastoma because the anterior portion of the pituitary gland arises from the ectoderm of the stomodeum. One of the clinical manifestations of hypopituitarism occurring in childhood is *dwarfism*. Since the essential changes of hypopituitarism occurring early in life are related to growth, abnormalities of eruption and crowding of teeth may occur.

Many studies of hormonal influence on body structures are carried out by removing the pituitary glands (hypophysectomy) of animals. Results are quite similar for all hypophysectomized animals and man. Complete removal of the pituitary gland in young animals results in a cessation of growth and failure of maturation of sex glands. In the adult animal there is atrophy of sex glands and organs, involution of thyroid, parathyroids, and adrenal cortex, and depression of their functions. Many disturbances also occur in the metabolism of carbohydrates, lipids, and proteins. Hypophysectomized animals are particularly sensitive to cold, infections, dietary deficiencies, stress, and insulin.

Although changes in the periodontium due to hypopituitarism occurring in hypophysectomized animals have been studied, changes typical of chronic destructive periodontal disease have not been demonstrated. Many evaluations of the effects of hypopituitarism on the periodontium do not consider the changes due to secondary effects related to other endocrine glands and the lowering of resistance to injury. The prevalence and severity of periodontal disease in human dwarfs do not appear to be different from that in the average population. The periodontal effects in patients with pituitary myxedema and panhypopituitarism are not clear, but there is no reason to suspect any particular or significant relationship between such disease states and periodontal disease. In effect, the periodontal changes associated with hypophysectomized animals do not parallel the histologic or clinical picture of chronic destructive periodontal disease seen in man.

Hyperpituitarism

The clinical manifestations of hyperpituitarism may be due to an overproduction of the growth hormone, adrenocorticotropic hormone, or even the thyrotropic hormone. However, the main effect of hyperpituitarism is an overgrowth of bones and connective tissue. As mentioned previously, the effect of pituitary gland disorders on all structures is related to the age at which a disturbance of functional activity occurs. If pituitary hyperfunction becomes apparent prior to the completion of ossification, then *giantism* results. However, if the hyperfunction occurs after ossification is completed, then *acromegaly* is the result.

The principal changes in acromegaly are enlargement of the terminal portions of the skeleton, hypertrophy of the connective tissue, and enlargement of the lips, tongue, hands, and feet. Because of an overgrowth of the connective tissue, the skin is thick and coarse, and often there is an increase in the amount of hair present. Since there is a continued overgrowth of bone at the terminal portions of the skeleton, the mandible becomes enlarged resulting in spacing of teeth and projection of the chin (prognathism). Except for the possibility of food impaction associated with the spacing of the teeth and mouth-breathing associated with prognathism, there is no indication that the prevalence and severity of chronic destructive periodontal disease or gingivitis are any greater in individuals with acromegaly than in normal individuals.

In *giantism* there is a general overgrowth of tissue so that the height of the afflicted individual may far exceed that of the range of normal individuals. Giantism is due to hyperplasia of the pituitary gland, and a tumor often is present involving the anterior lobe. In addition to an overgrowth of the skeleton, the clinical manifestations of pituitary insufficiency may also occur. Not infrequently the action of insulin is depressed and the symptoms of diabetes mellitus ensue. The dental structures are usually compatible with the size of the individual, and there are no known changes in the periodontium that can be attributed specifically to giantism.

In some instances, hyperpituitarism is due to a basophilic adenoma of the pituitary gland, which results in excessive production of ACTH and the manifestations of Cushing's syndrome. However, in most cases, Cushing's syndrome is related to disease of the adrenal cortex. However, whether Cushing's syndrome is produced by disease of the adrenal cortex or overproduction of ACTH, the clinical manifestations are the same and are discussed under disturbances of the adrenal glands.

ADRENAL DYSFUNCTION

The adrenal gland consists of a cortex and a medulla which are structurally and functionally different. The hormones (including cortisone, hydrocortisone, and aldosterone) of the adrenal cortex are steroids concerned with the control of water and electrolytes (mineralcorticoids), carbohydrate (glucocorticoids), protein and fat metabolism, and the sex hormones (androgens). The hormones (amines) of the medullary portion of the adrenal glands include epinephrine (adrenalin) and norepinephrine (noradrenalin). These hormones have an effect similar to that exerted by postganglionic fibers (adrenergic activity). Norepinephrine and epinephrine have similar effects, but norepinephrine is especially effective in constriction of arterioles and elevation of arterial blood pressure. Secretion of these hormones is controlled by the hypothalamus.

The mineralcorticoids influence cell permeability, especially renal cells, to various salts where excretion of potassium and retention of sodium are promoted. Aldosterone (or desoxycorticosterone), which represents the mineralcorticosteroids, provides the mechanism by which sodium, potassium, and extracellular fluids are maintained in normal balance. It should be pointed out that aldosterone secretion is independent of control by the anterior pituitary (ACTH) gland. Aside from functional disorders, hyperaldosteronism occurs in association with heart failure and hypertension. The loss of large amounts of sodium and the retention of potassium affect the cardiovascular and nervous systems to such an extent that life may not be possible.

The glucocorticoids, which are concerned with intermediate carbohydrate metabolism, include hydrocortisone and cortisone. These hormones are gluconeogenic in that they convert amino acids into sugar instead of into protein, resulting in increased blood sugar and glycogen in the liver. In addition to the influence on carbohydrate, protein, and fat metabolism, cortisone can suppress the inflammatory reaction of the tissues to many forms of irritation. Cortisone has been used in the treatment of painful symptoms of rheumatoid arthritis, but is of limited value in that the hormone does not influence the cause of the disease.

The sex hormones of the adrenal cortex are anabolic as well as androgenic in function. They are related to masculinization of the body, and tend to counteract the action of the glucocorticoids.

Hypoadrenalism (Hypocorticalism)

Although hypoadrenalism is essentially chronic in character, acute insufficiency occurs in certain circumstances, i.e., adrenal hemorrhage or extreme stress related to surgical operations, traumatic injuries, or acute illnesses.

The manifestation of chronic adrenal insufficiency is Addison's disease. The cause of adrenal insufficiency is usually tuberculosis, but it may be caused by other diseases such as hemorrhage, amyloidosis, and neoplasia; however, the cortex of both adrenal glands must be almost completely destroyed to produce an insufficiency. The manifestations of Addison's disease are general languor and debility, gastrointestinal irritation, loss of weight, craving for salt, low blood pressure, and increased pigmentation of skin and mucous membranes. The pigmentation of the hands, face, and neck gives a dingy hue to the skin, while dark spots may be found on the lips, tongue, gingiva, and buccal mucosa. Patients with Addison's disease react very poorly to traumatic experiences and surgery.

Adrenal insufficiency may be related to hypopituitarism and secondary to cortisone administration. Cortisone and related compounds produce a suppression of the pituitary as well as of the adrenal cortex. Perioral and oral pigmentation as well as other symptoms of adrenal insufficiency may ensue in such cases of secondary adrenal insufficiency.

Hyperadrenalism (Hyperadrenalcorticism)

Adrenocortical hyperfunction is usually due to either a tumor or bilateral hyperplasia of the cortices of the adrenal glands. The most characteristic manifestations of hyperfunction are Cushing's syndrome and the adrenogenital syndrome (adrenal virilism). The manifestations of Cushing's syndrome are due to excessive production of hydrocortisone by the adrenal cortex. The clinical manifestations are a peculiar, painful adiposity involving the face, neck, and trunk resulting in a moon-shaped face, "buffalo" or "bison" hump on the neck, and a protuberant abdomen. Other manifestations are hypertension, hirsutism in women and preadolescent boys, hyperglycemia and glycosuria, disturbances of sex function and psyche, muscular weakness, and a marked susceptibility to infection. The adrenogenital syndrome is produced by the presence of an excess of masculinizing (androgen) hormones. The clinical manifestations are dependent upon the sex of the patient, the age at onset, and the cause of the adrenal hyperfunction. However, in general, the clinical picture is characterized by virilism, hirsutism, and increased muscularity. In infants the great muscularity characterizes the picture of a miniature Hercules.

Stress and Disease

The relationship of the adrenal gland to stresses such as extreme heat or cold, and trauma has been studied rather extensively. It has been found that adrenalectomized animals have little ability to tolerate stresses such as extreme heat or cold, prolonged muscular activity, infections, intoxications, and other agents which increase the metabolic demands of the organism and stimulate adrenocortical function. Under continued stress, the pituitary-adrenal axis produces increased amounts of hormones to provide for the stress to the organism. Under these conditions of nonspecific stress, the tissues may respond to the hormonal stimulation by causing diseases called diseases of adaptation. While certain changes of the tissues occurring in animals as the result of synthetic hormonal imbalance and stress simulate human disease, they do not appear to be true diseases that can be related to normal subjects exposed to naturally occurring stresses. In this light, it is suggested that the role of the adrenal is a permissive one, i.e., the adrenal does not initiate the response but only allows a response to occur.

Periodontal changes in animals in the later stages of the stress syndrome include osteoporosis, reduction in the number of collagen fibers, degeneration of periodontal membrane, reduced osteoblastic activity, hemorrhage, and loss of supporting bone. Of paramount significance is the fact that periodontal pockets, which are characteristic of chronic destructive periodontal disease, have not been reported to occur under the laboratory conditions of stressing.

The idea that the connective tissues as a system may be injured by aberrations of the endocrine organs and that these injuries represent diseases of adaptation to the stress is not accepted with any firmness. The morphologic similarities of lesions in experimental animals to certain lesions in human diseases appear to be only superficial whether considering collagen diseases or periodontal disease. Even if the human and animal lesions were identical, such an identity in itself would not prove a unique cause.

THYROID DYSFUNCTION

The chief functions of the thyroid gland are to elaborate, store, and secrete a thyroid hormone (thyroxin) which is concerned mainly with the regulation of metabolic rate. In this respect, the thyroid hormones increase basal metabolism, are necessary for proper growth, are necessary for proper functioning of the nervous system, and, to some extent, affect cardiac metabolism and water and electrolyte balance. Thyroid dysfunction may be manifested by hypo- or hyperfunction of the thyroid glands.

Hypothyroidism

A deficiency of thyroid secretion may occur because the thyroid gland fails to develop properly during fetal life. The manifestations of hypothyroidism occurring in infancy are referred to as *cretinism*. The manifestations of hypothyroidism occurring at any time after early childhood are termed myxedema; however, myxedema usually is characteristic of the adult deficiency.

The primary features of cretinism are related to the lack of growth and mental and sexual development. There is a lack of growth of the long bones especially, although other bones, such as the mandible, maxilla, and the base of the skull, may also be underdeveloped. The head is large and the face broad with coarse features. In more severe cases, the tongue is thick and broad and the hair and skin dry because of atrophic sweat glands. In general, the temperature of the cretin is subnormal and his extremities are cold to touch. Dental development is slow and the eruption rate of the teeth is delayed with prolonged retention of the deciduous teeth. The dental age is below the chronologic age.

Juvenile myxedema is hypothyroidism occurring later in life than cretinism and is less severe. There is a lack of bone growth, cessation of mental development, and some skin changes. If the hypothyroidism begins during or after puberty, there are no changes in stature. While the other findings are similar to cretinism in juvenile myxedema they are much more variable and the manifestations may be overlooked in early stages of this disease.

In adult myxedema, the skin is dry and thickened and the lips are thickened. There is edema of the face and extremities, dry hair, thinning of the eyebrows, and enlargement of the lips, nose, tongue, and eyelids. An individual with myxedema often complains unduly of sensitivity to cold and has a low metabolic rate. There is no indication that wound healing is inadequate in these patients or that there is a direct relationship between hypothyroidism and periodontal disease or dental caries.

Hyperthyroidism

The most common form of hyperthyroidism is related to diffuse toxic or exophthalmic goiter, but also may be seen in association with a simple goiter. Hyperthyroidism is found most frequently after puberty and in women of childbearing age, but may occur at any age in both men and women. The clinical manifestations are variable, but most often include increased pulse rate and elevated blood pressure, irritability, intolerance to heat, sweating, tremor, loss of weight, prominence of the eyes (exophthalmus), tremor of hands and fingers, and muscular weakness.

In hyperthyroidism, osteoporosis may occur secondary to a loss of calcium and nitrogen. Such bone changes are not characteristic of chronic destructive periodontal disease and cannot be considered to be initiating factors in the development of periodontal disease. It has not been shown that osteoporosis appreciably influences the progress or severity of chronic destructive periodontal disease. There is some tendency for the primary teeth to be exfoliated earlier than normal and for the accelerated eruption of the permanent teeth. In animals with sever thyrotoxicosis, osteoporosis of the jaw, marrow fibrosis, degenerative changes of the principal fibers, and an increase in width of the periodontal membrane occur. As with the bone loss of hypothyroidism, the changes in the periodontium of experimental animals with severe hyperthyroidism are not analogous to the changes of chronic destructive periodontal disease with the production of pockets. Although hyperthyroidism may be a factor in the progress or severity of periodontal disease, it cannot be concluded that it is an initiating factor in periodontal disease.

Of significance is the possibility that patients with even mild hyperthyroidism may develop a thyroid crisis during surgical procedures or even during preparation for surgery. A thyroid crisis is characterized by a high fever, rapid heart rate, extreme nervousness, delirium, and, occasionally, coma. Such patients have an increased sensitivity to epinephrine in anesthetic solutions administered locally.

PARATHYROID DYSFUNCTION

The function of the parathyroid glands is to produce a hormone (parathormone) which controls calcium and phosphorus metabolism. Parathormone is important in the transference of calcium between the blood and the skeleton, controls the excretion of calcium and phosphate by the kidneys, and is an important factor in maintaining the excitability of the tissues and permeability of cell membranes. Because the parathyroid glands regulate the metabolism of calcium, phosphorus, and bone, there can be little question that these glands are important to calcification during the development of the supporting structures of the teeth, enamel and dentin, and to the maintenance of the supporting bone of the teeth and the entire skeleton. The action of parathormone increases the serum calcium and lowers the serum phosphorus. The increased level of calcium in the serum resulting from the action of the hormone is derived from the bones or from ingested calcium salts.

Hypoparathyroidism

A decrease in the secretion of parathormone may be due to various diseases, including neoplasms, or to accidental removal of the parathyroid glands at the time of thyroidectomy. The clinical manifestation of hypoparathyroidism is *tetany*. In tetany there is a marked drop in the blood calcium and increased neuromuscular irritability ensues. The manifestations of hypoparathyroidism include muscle cramps, aches and pains, convulsions, laryngeal spasms, dry scaly skin, frequent headaches, irritability, frequent association with thrush or candidiasis, and paresthesias (numbness and tingling sensations). It has been reported that an insufficient secretion of parathyroid hormone in infancy results in defective enamel formation (aplasia, hypoplasia) and blunting of the roots of the molar teeth.

Of interest are the manifestations of tetany owing to hyperventilation. Rapid, shallow, or hysterical over-breathing in emotional patients may lead to the manifestations of tetany without hypoparathyroidism. However, even slight hyperventilation may induce tetany in patients who have hypocalcemia and latent tetany related to hypocalcemia and hypoparathyroidism.

Hyperparathyroidism

Hypersecretion of the parathyroid hormone may result from neoplasms involving the parathyroid glands or from diffuse hyperplasia of the parathyroid glands. Hypersecretion may also result secondarily from hyperplasia of the parathyroid glands owing to calcium deprivation or renal disease. In the first instance, the dysfunction is called primary hyperparathyroidism; in the case of the compensatory response to a deficiency of calcium or to renal disease, the dysfunction is called secondary hyperparathyroidism.

The effects of hyperparathyroidism may be related to the musculoskeletal system and to the genitourinary system. Also involved less prominently is the gastrointestinal system. Musculoskeletal symptoms include localized or generalized pains in the bones, spontaneous fracture, tumors of the extremities and jaws, and bone deformities. Genitourinary symptoms include renal stones and infections secondary to obstruction by the stones, hematuria, renal insufficiency, and polyuria. Gastrointestinal symptoms include nausea, loss of weight, vomiting, constipation, and anorexia (loss of appetite).

The most prominent effect of hyperparathyroidism is decalcification of the bones, osteoporosis, and marked deformity of the bones. As the disease progresses and deformity of the bones develop, the disease is known as von Recklinghausen's disease of bone. In areas of decalcification, there is replacement of the bone by newly formed fibrous tissue with the production of small, pseudocystic lesions in bone; the process is termed *osteitis fibrosa cystica*. Fibroblastic replacement of bone may be accompanied by hemorrhage and numerous multinucleated giant cells producing a "brown tumor" which histologically is typical of hyperparathyroidism. Radiographically, the bone lesions appear to have a "ground-glass" appearance.

The occurrence of bone lesions involving the jaws may radiographically simulate ameloblastomas or other lesions, such as multiple myeloma and eosinophilic granuloma. Lesions of the jaw bones may suggest the periapical radiolucencies of periapical infection and the loss of lamina dura of the alveolar bone suggestive of chronic destructive periodontal disease. However, in the former instance the involved teeth are vital; in the latter, the loss of lamina dura is not related to the development of periodontal pockets. It is, of course, possible to have the lesions of periapical infection (periapical

19

radiolucencies) and periodontal disease concurrent with the lesions of hyperparathyroidism. Since periapical infection develops secondarily to pulp disease, the vitality of the teeth can be tested and related to carious lesions. Also, periodontal pockets develop only secondarily to the presence of irritating local factors such as calculus and dental plaque.

PANCREATIC HORMONE DYSFUNCTION

The principal endocrine disturbance related to the pancreas (*diabetes mellitus*) is not a disease of the pancreas, nor are there always observable lesions of the islands of Langerhans (the site of the production of the hormone, insulin). Diabetes mellitus is a disorder of carbohydrate metabolism characterized by a persistent hyperglycemia and often glycosuria and a deficiency of insulin. However, several processes are involved in diabetes mellitus, and a deficiency of insulin must be considered relative to the requirements of the tissues. Insulin makes possible the storage of glycogen in the liver and muscles; it enables the conversion of carbohydrate to fat, prevents the formation of sugar from protein in the liver, provides for oxidation of glucose by the peripheral tissues, and, in effect, participates in the regulation of blood sugar levels. However, the principal disturbance in diabetes mellitus appears to be related to an inability to store sugar as glycogen. Heredity, diet, obesity, and other endocrine gland dysfunctions are important in the etiology of diabetes mellitus.

The manifestations of fully developed diabetes mellitus include the accumulation of glucose in the blood (hyperglycemia); the excretion of the glucose in the urine (glycosuria), when the resorptive capacity of the kidney has been exceeded; and the frequent passing of water (polyuria). Because of depletion of glycogen stores in the liver, there is a conversion of protein to glucose and incomplete metabolism of fat. This disturbance results in the production of large quantities of ketone bodies. The production of ketone bodies results in ketosis leading to acidosis which, if untreated, causes coma and death. However, the principal clinical manifestations of diabetes usually are *polydipsia* (increased thirst), *polyphagia* (increased eating), and *polyuria* (increased urination).

There are several significant complications associated with uncontrolled diabetes. Diabetic individuals are particularly susceptible to infections, especially from staphylococcus and the tubercle bacillus organisms. Diabetics appear to be susceptible to abscess formation, carbuncles, tuberculosis, pneumonia, urinary tract infections, and multiple periodontal abscesses. They often have disturbances of the peripheral nervous system with widespread polyneuritis, numbness, and loss of pain sensation in the lower extremities, and occasionally mental changes. Accelerated arteriosclerosis is a major complication in patients with uncontrolled diabetes with chronic ulcers and diabetic gangrene frequently involving the lower extremities. Additional complications include retinal changes so that vision is severely impaired. Renal failure owing to arteriosclerosis is a common cause of death in the diabetic individual.

The possibility of diabetic acidosis, coma, and insulin reaction may be minimized with a proper schedule of eating and insulin injection prior to surgical procedures. Hyperinsulinism, resulting from an overdosage of the hormone, is characterized by nervousness, weakness, depression, cold sweats, confusion, anxiety, delirium, and, in severe cases, is followed by convulsions and collapse.

Aside from the possibility of the complication of infection following such procedures as the extraction of teeth, deep scaling, and gingivectomy, there is little evidence to indicate that healing following gingivectomy is significantly delayed even in the patient with uncontrolled diabetes. Periodontal abscesses and infection can and do occur after scaling of the teeth and periodontal surgery in patients with poorly controlled diabetes. In general, diabetics with good control of the disease are good candidates for periodontal therapy, deep scaling, and routine prophylaxis; however, patients with poorly controlled diabetes and periodontal disease may require more conservative treatment, antibiotic coverage, and careful attention following any surgical or scaling procedure. Aside from the patient receiving no treatment, a patient with poorly controlled diabetes is one who has progressive manifestations of diabetes even though under treatment, i.e., the patient is taking insulin and is eating properly, but has a chronic or progressive history of multiple periodontal abscesses, carbuncles, ulcers of the lower extremities, hypertension, and a poor periodontal response to adequate elimination of local irritating factors.

GONADAL DYSFUNCTION

The testes and ovaries produce hormones which control secondary sex characteristics, the reproductive cycle, and the growth and development of accessory reproductive organs. Testosterone is the principal naturally occurring male hormone and the chief androgen of the testis. The two principal hormones of the ovary are the follicular hormone (estradiol) and luteal hormone (progesterone). The estrogenic hormones are produced by the graffian follicles; the progestational hormones are derived from the corpus luteum of the ruptured follicles in the ovary. Gonadal dysfunction in both men and women may be due to failure of the pituitary gland to stimulate the gonads or adrenal glands, or to dysfunction of the gonads.

Hypogonadism

The effects of hypogonadism in men depend upon the age at onset of the disturbance. When there is a complete loss of testicular function as the result of inflammation, surgery, injury, or other causes before sex maturation takes place, secondary sex characteristics fail to appear. There is increased height due to prolonged growth of the lower extremities, producing a disproportionate length of the lower extremities to that of the trunk of the body. Such individuals are called eunuchs and the disturbance *eunuchism*. Testicular insufficiency following puberty and the development of the sex characteristics results in very little change in body structure. *Eunuchoidism* is a term usually used when referring to a partial loss of testicular function. In the presence of a pituitary deficiency of gonadotropin and other pituitary hormones, dwarfism and hypogonadal changes may result if the pituitary deficiency occurs prior to puberty.

Prepubertal hypogonadism in women may occur as the result of hypoplasia or absence of the gonads. When hypoplasia is the cause, there is an overgrowth of the long bones. In the absence of ovaries, growth is interfered with and dwarfism results. *Postpubertal hypogonadism* may result in hypoplasia of the sex organs, loss of secondary sex characteristics, and amenorrhea. Hypogonadism may be related directly to ovarian insufficiency or may be secondary to a deficiency of gonadotropic hormone secretion by the anterior pituitary gland.

The principal effects of ovarian insufficiency are amenorrhea, menopausal symptoms, hot flushes, gain in weight, sweating, nervous tension, and, less frequently, osteoporosis and hirsutism. Naturally occurring ovarian insufficiency between the ages of 45 and 50 years is the *menopause*. The symptoms of the menopause are numerous and include irregularity and cessation of the menses, emotional disturbances, arthralgia, fatigue, hot flushes, sweating, and headaches. Hirsutism and osteoporosis are not uncommon. As indicated in Chapter 11 on periodontal disease, some forms of gingivitis have been secondarily related to hormonal imbalance during and following menopause (p. 235). Secondary ovarian insufficiency is related to a disturbance of gonadotropin secretion by the pituitary gland and to the action of the hypothalamus on the pituitary.

Hypergonadism

Some tumors of the testes result in the overproduction of gonadal hormones. The manifestations of hypergonadism vary with the age at onset.

Prepubertal hypergonadism associated with an overgrowth of the testes tends to result in precocious puberty and premature development of all male sex characteristics. *Postpubertal hypergonadism,* following the completion of skeletal development, results in few changes; under some circumstances feminization may take place.

An overproduction of ovarian hormones may result in abnormal menstrual changes. It must be recognized that relative hypergonadism is very common during the active reproductive period and is usually of no importance. However, uterine bleeding prior to puberty and after menopause may be due to neoplasms. Prepubertal hypergonadism results in precocious puberty with premature onset of menses, secondary sex characteristics, and rapid skeletal growth. In some instances, such hypergonadism is due to tumors of the ovaries. Postpubertal hypergonadism may be primary or secondary in origin and is characterized primarily by changes in the menstrual cycle.

A few ovarian neoplasms are functional and give rise to masculinization, feminization, or precocious puberty and menstrual bleeding.

BIBLIOGRAPHY

Harrison, T. R. (Ed.): Principles of Internal Medicine. New York, McGraw-Hill Book Co., 1966.

Kupperman, H. S.: Human Endocrinology. Philadelphia, F. A. Davis Co., 1963.

MacKenzie, R. S., and Millard, H. D.: Interrelated effects of diabetes, arteriosclerosis and calculus on alveolar bone loss. J. Amer. Dent. Ass., 66:191, 1963.

O'Leary, T. M., Shannon, I., and Prigmore, J. R.: Clinical and systemic findings in periodontal disease. J. Periodont., 33:243, 1962.

Selye, H.: The general adaptation syndrome and the diseases of adaptation. J. Clin. Endocr., 6:117, 1946.

The blood, even though fluid in character, is a tissue. It is composed of several types of cells with a wide range of functions. While other tissues and organs have their parenchymal cells fixed into a histologic pattern, the blood has a fluid matrix and circulates throughout the body. The formative elements of the blood are contained in the bone marrow and the lymphoid tissue. The bone marrow and lymphoid tissue comprise the hemopoietic system which produces the blood cells. In blood dyscrasias, attention has to be given to the formative tissues because they are the seat of the disease, whereas peripheral blood is the product reflecting the nature of the alterations in the formative organ. Many blood dyscrasias are named for the changes in the peripheral blood.

COMPONENTS OF BLOOD

The blood is composed of a number of elements and alterations in all elements must be considered. The components of the blood are blood plasma, red blood cells, white blood cells, platelets or thrombocytes, and other factors involved in blood coagulation. These components of the blood show both physiologic and pathologic alterations which are reflections of disease in the hemopoietic system or as the result of disease in some other area of the body.

Blood plasma is a complex saline fluid containing numerous complex proteins of large molecular size designated albumins and globulins. The globulins include antibodies, which protect the individual against infection, and fibrinogen and other clotting factors, such as factors V, VII, IX, and X. Other plasma proteins, such as prothrombin, are albumins and are essential for blood clotting. They are present in the blood as fibrinogen and are precipitated from extravasated blood to form fibrin which entraps both red and white blood cells to form blood clots that inhibit hemorrhage. Alterations occur in the plasma proteins and result in disease processes.

The *red blood cells* are biconcave discs 9 μ (microns) in diameter that are filled with hemoglobin, an iron-containing substance, which has a marked affinity for oxygen that is responsible for its transportation. Red blood cells are produced by the bone marrow and expelled into the peripheral blood to maintain a constant level in the number of cells, or they are produced in greater number to meet the demand for greater oxygen-carrying capacity. The individual who lives at a high altitude or who has lung disease with decreased respiratory capacity has a larger number of red blood cells in the peripheral blood than a normal individual living at sea level. Normally there are 4 to 5.5 million red blood cells per cu. mm. of blood, but in individuals living at high altitudes the red cells increase by a million or more per cu. mm. of blood. There is also a physiologic increase in the number of cells per cu. mm. in dehydration. The red blood cells decrease in number when the iron intake is low or when there is massive hemorrhage, viz., after a blood loss of 1000 cu. mm. there would be an appreciable temporary reduction in blood cells per cu. mm. In addition to the physiologic alterations in the number of red blood cells, there are pathologic alterations to be discussed later.

The *white blood cells* (leukocytes) are of three types: neutrophils (PMN's, granulocytes), lymphocytes, and large mononuclear cells (monocytes). Normally there are 7 to 9 thousand leukocytes per cu. mm. of blood. The polymorphonuclear leukocyte (PMN) is a white blood cell formed by the bone marrow and maintained in the peripheral blood at a constant level. They make up about 65 percent of the white blood cells in the peripheral blood. These cells are the first line of defense in inflammation and protect against infection (p. 73). When injury occurs, there is a demand for a greater number of cells in the area of injury, so more are expelled from the bone marrow increasing the number in the peripheral blood. The physiologic increase is called *leukocytosis* and, in addition to resulting from infection, occurs during pregnancy, dehydration, exposure, following ingestion of a big meal, and cyclically every 12 hours. The white blood cells may also decrease in number physiologically. This condition is called *leukopenia* and occurs in relation to some chemical substances, starvation, and shock.

The *lymphocytes* constitute about 40 percent of the white blood cells in the peripheral circulation. They are formed in the lymph nodes and the other areas of the body containing lymphoid tissue and are expelled into the lymph fluid which carries them to the blood stream. The increase of lymphocytes in the peripheral blood is termed *lymphocytosis* and occurs with some infections (especially viral infections), chronic tuberculosis, and as a relative process in neutropenia. Lymphopenia may result from starvation and be relative to granulocytosis.

The *large mononuclear cells* are produced by the reticuloendothelial system which resides in the bone marrow, lymphoid tissue, and some of the viscera (liver and lung). The monocytes are the fewest in number of the white blood cells making up only about 8 to 10 percent of the total. This group of cells demonstrates less physiologic fluctuation than the other leukocytes, but increase in number in some infections such as typhoid fever, chronic tuberculosis, and in response to chemical toxicity. Reduction in the number of monocytes is uncommon but may occur in response to some chemical toxicity.

Another cellular element of the blood is the *thrombocyte* or *platelet*. Platelets are products of the bone marrow and are present in the peripheral blood to participate in the blood-clotting mechanism. The platelets vary in number from 200,000 to 500,000 per cu. mm. of blood and do not show physiologic alterations, but may be altered in disease. They may, however, be reduced in toxic alteration of the bone marrow, but in this instance the thrombocytopenia results in hemorrhagic disease.

Composition of the Blood
(Adult Male)

Plasma—3 to 4 liters
Red blood cells—4 to 5.5 million per cu. mm. of blood
Hemoglobin—12.5 to 16 Gm. per 100 ml. of blood
(higher in men than in women)
White blood cells—7 to 9,000 per cu. mm. of blood
Platelets—200 to 300 thousand per cu. mm. of blood

Normal White Cell Values
(% of Total)

Neutrophils (granulocytes)—45 to 65 percent
Lymphocytes—25 to 40 percent
Large mononuclear cells—8 to 10 percent
Eosinophils—2 to 4 percent
Basophils—0 to 1 percent

PLASMA ALTERATIONS

Hypofibrinogenemia is an acquired or congenital disease characterized by a reduction in the quantity of fibrinogen in the peripheral blood. The reduced amount of fibrinogen results in an increased bleeding time due to delayed clotting because of a lack of fibrin. Gingival bleeding is a characteristic of this rare disease. The acquired lack of fibrinogen may be due to liver disease, extensive hemorrhage both acute and chronic, transfusion reaction, polycythemia, certain neoplasms, and pregnancy.

Macroglobulinemia is a disease caused by the increase in size and numbers of the plasma globules. The patients usually have anemia and increased viscosity of the blood. Patients are most often men over 50 years of age who are pale, weak, with marked loss of weight. Bleeding occurs from the gums and nose as well as in the central nervous system.

A reduction in quantity of plasma and electrolytes occurs with significant loss of blood, high temperature, and a reduction in fluid intake, which is associated with increased viscosity and other manifestations of dehydration.

BLOOD CELL ALTERATIONS

Disease states occur both with increased or decreased numbers of various types of blood cells. As indicated in the following outline, the alteration of numbers of cells is given a name. The upper term indicates an excess of cells and the lower term a decrease of cells.

Designation for Alteration of Blood Elements

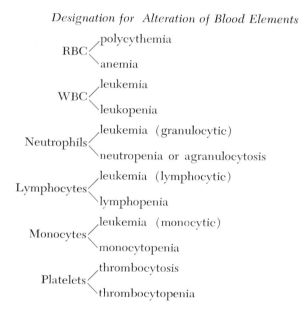

```
              ╱polycythemia
      RBC ⟨
              ╲anemia

              ╱leukemia
      WBC ⟨
              ╲leukopenia

                  ╱leukemia  (granulocytic)
   Neutrophils ⟨
                  ╲neutropenia or agranulocytosis

                  ╱leukemia  (lymphocytic)
  Lymphocytes ⟨
                  ╲lymphopenia

               ╱leukemia  (monocytic)
   Monocytes ⟨
               ╲monocytopenia

              ╱thrombocytosis
   Platelets ⟨
              ╲thrombocytopenia
```

Red Blood Cells

Polycythemia loosely refers to an increase in number of red blood cells (erythrocytes). It may be compensatory due to a lowered oxygen-carrying capacity of the blood which is compensated for by an increase in the number of red blood cells (erythrocytosis). It may also refer to a pathologic increase in the red blood cells due to a disease of the bone marrow with extra red cells being expelled into the peripheral blood (erythremia, polycythemia rubra vera).

Aplastic anemia is characterized by a decrease in all bone marrow elements, including red blood cells, platelets, and granulocytes. It may be produced by the action of toxic agents on the bone marrow causing a severe, progressive, and always fatal anemia with purpuric and hemorrhagic phenomena present in the later stages. Aplastic anemia may be primary in type due to hereditarily induced bone marrow alterations.

Hemolytic anemias are characterized by an increased destruction of red blood cells. Hereditary hemolytic anemias include sickle cell anemia and thalassemia as well as others. Acquired hemolytic anemias include those due to drugs and infection and erythroblastosis fetalis.

In *sickle cell anemia* the red blood cells have a sickle shape, giving the disease its name. It occurs almost exclusively in Negroes. Manifestations include episodes of muscle, joint, and abdominal pains and neurologic disorders. Orally, there is evidence of bone changes produced by increase in size of marrow spaces and loss of bone trabeculae. Because of proliferation of marrow, there is an increase in size of alveolar process with spacing of the teeth. The alveolar bone (lamina dura) is not affected.

Thalassemia (Cooley's anemia, Mediterranean disease) is a chronic progressive hemolytic anemia characterized by increased destruction of red blood cells. It is seen in people of Mediterranean, African, and Asian ancestry as well as in people living in the Mediterranean basin. In the severe form of the disease, there is severe anemia, atypical nucleated red cells, and skeletal changes. The onset is within the first or second year of life causing the child to have a yellow pallor, fever, chills, malaise, and generalized weakness. The child's features are often mongoloid due to changes in the maxillary facial and cranial bones. There is osteoporosis with bone marrow hyperplasia, which is responsible for the bone changes and an associated spacing of teeth. Intraoral radiographs show a pattern of bone similar to that seen in sickle cell anemia. The oral mucosa demonstrates the pallor and mild icteric tint seen in other forms of anemia.

Erythroblastosis fetalis is a congenital hemolytic anemia due to sensitization of a pregnant Rh-negative woman by Rh agglutinating factors from her Rh-positive fetus. In effect, there is an incompatibility between maternal and fetal blood factors. When the mother is Rh-negative and the father Rh-positive, the fetus inherits the paternal factor, which may act as an antigen to the mother, immunizing her with the production of antibodies that, when transferred back to the fetus through the placenta, initiate hemolysis of fetal blood. The hemolytic process may cause prenatal death with miscarriage, or it may be manifest at birth as icterus and progressive hemolytic disease of the newborn. Because of the intense hemolysis from the formation of abundant bile pigment, icterus develops that may cause teeth in the process of forming to show mild hypoplasia and pigmentation of enamel and dentin. Such intrinsic staining gives the teeth a greenish-brown hue.

White Blood Cells

Blood diseases may involve disturbances of the white blood cells. The alteration of white blood cells may be physiologic and occur in response to processes which require alteration in number or type of cells. The white blood cells are a necessary part of the defense mechanism and increase in number during inflammation. The type and extent of increase in white cells are influenced by the extent and nature of the injury. Granulocytes increase in response to coccal infections; lymphocytes increase in response to viral infections. The increase in white cells as a part of the inflammatory response is physiologic and is called leukocytosis.

Leukemia is a pathologic increase in white blood cells due to neoplastic processes in hemopoietic tissue resulting in an increase of abnormal cells in the peripheral blood. A decrease in the number of white blood cells may be due to depressed activity of the bone marrow by toxins, infection of the bone marrow, the replacement of the bone marrow by another tissue, or to a nutritional deficiency. A general reduction of white blood cells is called *leukopenia;* a reduction of polymorphonuclear cells is *granulocytopenia* or *neutropenia;* a reduction of monocytes is *monocytopenia;* and a reduction of lymphocytes is *lymphopenia* or *lymphocytopenia*. *Granulocytopenia* or *neutropenia* usually refers to a physiologic decrease in white cells, whereas *agranulocytosis* or *malignant neutropenia* indicates a pathologic decrease with severe depressant action on leukocyte formation and with very few cells in the peripheral blood.

The most common form of *agranulocytosis* is due to the depressant action of drugs and bacterial toxins. Any drug which is toxic to a person or to which the individual has a hypersensitivity may cause hypofunction of bone marrow. Amidopyrine is the most common offender, but all drugs containing the benzine ring as a part of their molecular structure may produce the disease. Dinitrophenol, thiouracil, sulfonamides, arsenicals, thorazine, and quinidine are some of the common offenders. The disease is most common in the population who uses drugs, so professional personnel have the highest incidence of the disease. The incidence is about two to three times more common in women than in men. Shortly after ingestion of the drug, the bone marrow is depressed and the white cells disappear from the peripheral blood. The individual has an elevation in temperature, general malaise, fatigue, and a sore throat. The symptoms progress rapidly to become severe and death ensues within a few days to a week. Ulcerations develop in the mouth and throat, providing a pathway for invasion of organisms to which the individual has no resistance due to lack of white blood cells (Fig. 162). The developing bacteremia and septicemia cause death. The disease was fatal in 95 percent of patients before antibiotics were available and even with heavy antibiotic therapy the disease is fatal in 50 percent of the individuals having the disease.

Agranulocytosis may be secondary to leukemia in which the bone marrow is replaced by neoplastic tissue and white cells are not produced. The signs and symptoms of the disease are the same as for leukemia but are less dramatic in occurrence and effect. The disease is nonetheless fatal. The termination of the leukemic patient is often on the basis of agranulocytosis.

Leukemia is due to a neoplasm of hemopoietic tissue in which the neoplastic cells appear in the peripheral blood. *Myelogenous leukemia* occurs when the bone marrow is the site of the neoplasm and the granulocytic series of cells is involved. *Lymphatic* or *lymphoid leukemia* occurs when the neoplasm (lymphoblastoma or lympho-

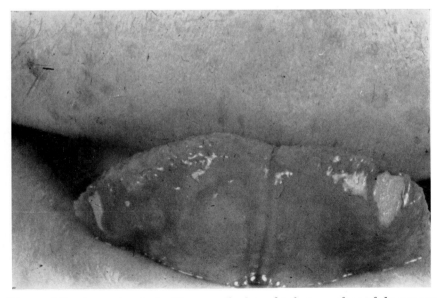

Figure 162. *Agranulocytosis.* Ulcers on the lateral inferior surface of the tongue have rolled borders and are surfaced by a white membrane. There is a limited peripheral inflammatory reaction.

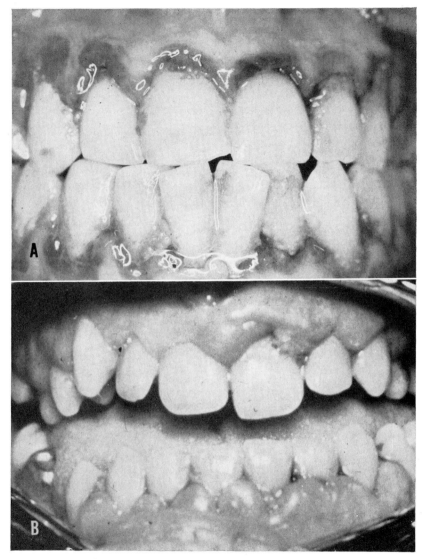

Figure 163. *Leukemia*. A, Marked marginal gingivitis in a patient with myelogenous leukemia. The gingival margins are highly colored, soft,
friable, and bleed easily. Abundant materia alba is evident. Inability to brush the teeth permits the accumulation of debris which
enhances the gingival disease. B, Typical hyperplasia of gingiva
with thick margins and bulbous interdental papillae. Interproximal necrosis and spontaneous hemorrhage into the embrasure
occurs.

sarcoma) involves lymphoid tissue and the neoplastic lymphocytes are found in the peripheral blood. When the reticuloendothelial elements found in both marrow and lymphoid tissue are
involved, *monocytic leukemia* is the result. The white cell count is
very high in leukemia, but the cells are neoplastic and do not
function as normal cells. The bone marrow is replaced by the neoplastic cells so that red blood cells and platelets are not formed and
the individual develops a secondary anemia and thrombocytopenia.
Leukemia may be acute or chronic depending upon the rate of
progress of the disease, but all types progress relentlessly to fatal
termination. All types of leukemia produce similar signs and symptoms with the same terminal findings.

The oral lesions of leukemia have the same characteristics for all
types of leukemia. There is gingival enlargement of rapid and
extensive occurrence with the tissue being soft, discolored, and
showing necrosis and spontaneous hemorrhage (Fig. 163A and B).
The gingival changes are progressive owing to the lack of resistance
to infection. The necrosis, which is often typical of necrotizing
ulcerative gingivitis (Vincent's infection), initiates hemorrhages that
are severe and often impossible to control. The intensity of the
gingival response is related to the state of gingival health which
existed at the onset of leukemia. Ulcerations in the mouth and
throat occur and progress extensively with the progress of the disease. The intense secondary anemia is also contributory to death,
as is the septicemia which often occurs.

Platelets

The platelets or thrombocytes produced by the bone marrow play
an active part in the clotting of blood. The platelets break down
when the blood is extravasated and liberate thromboplastin which
plays a part in the precipitation of fibrin to form the blood clot.
The absence of platelets or an alteration in their fragility results in
a tendency for hemorrhage into the tissues and is designated *thrombocytopenic purpura*. Purpura may be caused by aplastic disease
of the bone marrow as either a primary process or a process secondary to the action of drugs, leukemia, liver disease, vitamin C
deficiency, or the administration of anticoagulants as a therapeutic
procedure. Purpuras occur in leukemia because of the replacement
of bone marrow by neoplastic tissue and they are a frequent complication of the disease.

The aplastic type of purpura is called primary or idiopathic
thrombocytopenic purpura and is due to the inability of the bone
marrow to produce platelets, although other blood elements are unaffected. The patient bleeds freely and spontaneously into skin

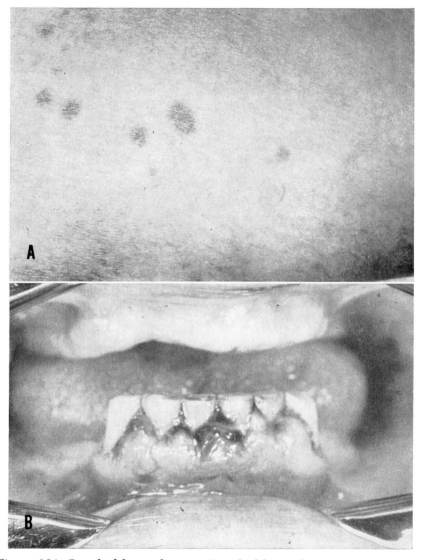

Figure 164. *Petechial hemorrhage.* A, Petechial hemorrhage in the skin of the arm of a patient having thrombocytopenic purpura secondary to leukemia. B, Hemorrhage from the crevicular zone and into the gingiva is typical, especially in the presence of subgingival calculus.

(Fig. 164A) and mucous membranes. The subcutaneous or mucosal hemorrhages are initiated by trauma, are manifested as petechiae or ecchymosis, and may result in massive hemorrhage. The degree of bleeding is dependent upon the severity of the trauma. In patients with gingival disease, gingival bleeding presents an early and difficult symptom to control. The bleeding from the gingiva may be of such intensity and duration as to require transfusions.

The changes in the gingiva caused by purpura are those of spontaneous bleeding or intense bleeding with minor trauma (Fig. 164B). The presence of tartar in the gingival sulcus initiates bleeding and in the presence of purpura the hemorrhage is continuous and severe. The bleeding may be intensified by scaling and always presents a problem with extraction of teeth. Even though bleeding may be intensified by scaling, the elimination of the calculus may alleviate the gingival hemorrhage. Bleeding occurs into joints, especially weight-bearing joints, producing a hemorrhagic arthritis; there is no significant involvement of the temporomandibular joints.

BLOOD COAGULATION FACTORS

There are at least 12 factors involved in the coagulation of blood. While a deficiency of some of the factors results in clearly definable blood dyscrasias in which there is a failure of hemostasis, some of the functions of the other factors are not clearly understood, nor are the manifestations of their deficiences readily apparent. The following table indicates the factors by number and name.

Blood Coagulation Factors

Factor	Name
I	Fibrinogen
II	Prothrombin
III	Thromboplastin
IV	Calcium
V	Labile factor
VI	(No longer designated)
VII	Stabile factor
VIII	Antihemophilic factor
IX	Christmas factor
X	Stuart-Prower factor
XI	Plasma thromboplastin antecedent
XII	Hageman factor

Such factors are "trace" proteins, except for calcium, and are in the blood in such small amounts that their presence is established indirectly and through genetic and biochemical tests. *Fibrinogen* is a plasma protein that is acted upon by thrombin to form fibrin.

Prothrombin is a precursor of thrombin that is produced by the liver. *Thromboplastin* has been referred to as the direct activator of prothrombin and may be found in the tissues, plasma, and platelets. *Calcium* in an ionized form is required for coagulation, but a deficiency sufficient to interfere with coagulation would be incompatible with life. The *labile factor* appears to be necessary for the formation of a prothrombin-converting substance. The *stabile factor* accelerates the conversion of prothrombin to thrombin in the presence of factors III, IV, and V. The *antihemophilic factor* is essential for blood thromboplastin formation. The *Christmas factor* is active in the formation of blood thromboplastin. Factor X influences the amount of plasma thromboplastin. Factor XI is concerned with the activation of plasma thromboplastin. Factor XII is related in some way to the clotting of the blood when in contact with glass tubes, but its precise role in coagulation is unknown.

The process of blood hemostasis is a very complex process and any simplified explanation is subject to many exceptions and limitations. The following discussion is not intended to be complete or to explain all of the various processes involved in the natural control of hemorrhage.

When a blood vessel is cut, there is an outflow of blood platelets which release several factors involved in the coagulation process and the constriction of blood vessels. In the latter, it is assumed that serotonin is responsible for the vasoconstriction and, to some extent, a drop in blood pressure, both processes tending to control the vascular elements of the hemorrhage as coagulation proceeds.

With the rupture of platelets and tissue injury, there is a release of thromboplastin which, in the presence of calcium and factors V, VII, VIII, IX, and X, activates prothrombin. The prothrombin is converted to thrombin which acts on fibrinogen to form fibrin. The fibrin strands become entangled with the formed elements of the blood including platelets which agglutinate to form a clot.

Since prothrombin is produced by the liver, diseases of the liver or obstructive jaundice results in hemorrhagic disease. The presence of anticoagulants, such as the antiprothrombins used in heart disease, inhibit the action of prothrombin and the tendency to bleed results (Fig. 165). A deficiency of prothrombin (hypoprothrombinemia) may be the result of a lack of vitamin K due to the obstruction of bile flow, impaired absorption, and the prolonged use of antibiotics which inhibit the growth of intestinal microorganisms. A deficiency may be related to a congenital deficiency of factor V and to factor VII. The deficiency may result in prolonged bleeding from the gingiva as well as the nose and other areas following surgery.

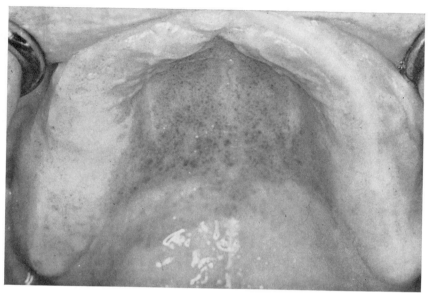

Figure 165. *Petechial hemorrhage.* Multiple petechial hemorrhages in the palate and on the crest of the ridge in a denture patient receiving anticoagulant therapy. The hemorrhage is extensive because of the negative pressure produced by the denture.

Hemophilia is a rare hereditary abnormality of blood that exhibits an intense bleeding problem. The disorder is a sex-linked recessive disease transmitted by women but exhibited by the men. The defect in coagulation is due to the absence or reduction of factor VIII, which is essential for the formation of blood thromboplastin. The disease is congenital and presents a problem throughout life because of the tendency for hemorrhage with minor trauma. The shedding of deciduous teeth or the extraction of teeth may lead to severe uncontrolled hemorrhage. A form of hemophilia called hemophilia B or *Christmas disease* is related to a deficiency of factor IX and the bleeding manifestations are usually less severe than in hemophilia.

In addition to an absence of clotting factors as a cause of bleeding, vascular defects may be responsible for hemorrhage. Bleeding that is difficult to control may be due to fragility and hyperelasticity of the investing tissues as seen in purpura senilis, Cushing's syndrome, and the Ehlers-Danlos syndrome. Prolonged vitamin C deficiency may result in bleeding of the gingiva and joints. The most common cause of gingival bleeding is related to gingivitis and periodontitis. Sometimes prolonged bleeding occurs following the scaling of teeth.

Most often such hemorrhage is related to the traumatic injury of vessels emerging from nutrient channels very close to the base of deep periodontal pockets. With the common administration of anticoagulants in "coronary" heart disease therapy, it is always essential to determine whether or not a patient has a potential or real bleeding tendency prior to scaling or surgical procedures. A short history of the patient's medical and dental backgrounds should provide sufficient evidence, in most instances, to rule out blood dyscrasias.

BIBLIOGRAPHY

Cohen, D. W., and Morris, A. L.: Periodontal manifestations of cyclic neutropenia. J. Periodont., 32:159, 1961.

Gates, A. F.: Chronic neutropenia presenting with oral lesions. Oral Surg., 27:563, 1969.

Gorlin, R. J., and Chaudry, A. P.: Oral manifestations of cyclic neutropenia. Arch. Derm. (Chicago), 82:344, 1960.

Krivit, W., and White, J. G.: A simplified approach for the detection of coagulation disorders. J. Lancet, 85:381, 1965.

Lewis, J. H.: Coagulation defects. J.A.M.A., 178:1014, 1961.

Lynch, M. A., and Ship, I. I.: Initial oral manifestations of leukemia. J. Amer. Dent. Ass., 75:938, 1967.

Spaet, T. H.: Hemorrhagic diseases: mechanisms and management. Hosp. Pract., 2:36, 1967.

Stohlman, F. J.: Erythropoiesis. New Eng. J. Med., 267:242, 1962.

White, G. E.: Oral manifestations of leukemia in children. Oral Surg., 29:420, 1970.

• Index

Page numbers in *italics* denote figures.

21
⨍